Blueprints for Your Bottom Line Series

Blueprints for Your Bottom Line

Dentistry: Creating a Profit Center

Coralee Eisner, CVT, MBA

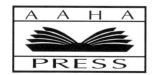

© 1999 AAHA Press
12575 W. Bayaud Avenue
Lakewood, CO 80228
800/252-2242 or 303/986-2800

ISBN 1-58326-004-8

Contents

Figures

Tables

Preface

In the fall of 1997, I was invited by the American Animal Hospital Association (AAHA) to write a guidebook to help practitioners with the business aspects of establishing a profitable dental department. Because most veterinarians receive relatively little business training, the purpose of this book is to guide the reader through the steps necessary to develop a dental profit center. The guidebook is designed to be used as a source for basic financial analysis, finding educational opportunities, designing and equipping a dental suite, and marketing dental services for all levels of practice, but primarily for those veterinarians wishing to raise their level of practice who are just beginning their advanced dental education.

I have been involved in veterinary practice for more than 20 years. After graduating from Colorado State University with a degree in economics, I worked as a statistician and computer programmer for Standard and Poor's, a subsidiary of McGraw-Hill. After meeting my future husband, Edward R. Eisner, DVM, I became interested in veterinary medicine and changed careers, earning an associate degree from Bel-Rea Institute of Animal Technology. In 1977, I joined the Campus Veterinary Clinic in Denver as a Certified Veterinary Technician and worked in that capacity for 10 years while also growing into the role of practice manager. I completed a master of business administration at the University of Colorado at Denver in 1995.

Beginning in 1982, my husband became interested in advanced veterinary dentistry as a way of providing better service to our clients and protecting the practice from the loss of business resulting from emerging vaccination and spay/neuter clinics. He became a diplomate of the American Veterinary Dental College in 1989 and operates the Denver Veterinary Dental Service, a referral dental specialty practice serving the Rocky Mountain region.

Throughout this book I use the example of a hypothetical veterinary hospital to illustrate the financial impact that a marketing program might have on a practice. I employ numbers that are representative of an average veterinary hospital in the United States. I used articles from *AAHA TRENDS Magazine, Veterinary Economics,* and various studies produced by AAHA as my sources. I have attempted to keep the examples basic and to be consistent in the numbers used to illustrate the key points.

It is important to be aware that numbers can be manipulated to show various results, but I believe you will find that the basic principles will hold true, regardless of the numbers used in the illustrations.

It is my hope that this book will be useful and informative and provide a few "golden nuggets" along the way. My goal is to aid my reader in leading his or her practice to greater success by providing high-quality dental care.

Coralee Eisner, CVT, MBA

Acknowledgments

Accepting a writing assignment is a great commitment of time and energy on the part of the author, with contributions and sacrifices made by the author's family. I would like to thank my husband, Ed Eisner, and daughter, Heather, for their support and understanding during the year that I was working on this project. I would also like to thank my husband for reviewing this book for technical errors and providing creative and other helpful suggestions. His input was invaluable. I also wish to thank my mother, Naoma O'Neill, a retired high school English teacher, for reviewing the book for grammatical correctness and clearness. They were a terrific support team.

In addition, I would like to thank the following diplomates of the American Veterinary Dental College for their input on facility design and their support of the project: Jan Bellows, DVM; Gregg DuPont, DVM; Steven Holmstrom, DVM; Thomas Kavanagh, DVM; Ken Lyon, DVM; Tom Mulligan, DVM; Frank Verstraete, DVM; and Robert Wiggs, DVM. I believe that their response to my questions added value to the guide. I would also like to thank Robert D. Chaney, DVM, of Pharmacia and Upjohn, for providing me with marketing materials, and Shor-Line/Schroer Manufacturing, Suburban Surgical, Summit Hill Laboratories, and Dentalaire for the photographs used in Chapter 5.

Finally, I would like to thank Mary Kay Kozyra, acquisitions editor for AAHA Press, and Dr. Bob Froehlich for offering me this opportunity and supporting me through the process.

Personal Anecdote: Dr. Ed Eisner first began performing advanced level dental care at the Campus Veterinary Clinic in 1983 with the help of Peter Emily, DDS, one of the innovators in the field of veterinary dentistry. I was also employed at the clinic, and at first I wasn't convinced that this level of dentistry was really necessary until I met Ozzie. He was a very large two-year-old mastiff with an unpleasant disposition, and both the client and referring veterinarian were afraid of Ozzie. He was referred for root canal therapy of a fractured tooth. After he was anesthetized, it was noticed that his lower canine teeth were positioned too far medially and were perforating his hard palate on both sides. While he was under anesthesia, Drs. Emily and Eisner lowered the length of the crowns of the two canines and placed a filling in the exposed root chamber. Ozzie recovered uneventfully and was discharged. When Dr. Eisner telephoned the owner two days later for a progress report, she stated that Ozzie was a new dog. His nasty temperament was gone and he had become a sweet and lovable family pet overnight. She was very grateful for the services our staff had performed. Ozzie had been in intolerable pain for most of his life until this simple dental treatment. This case turned me instantly into a believer. I have never doubted the importance of dental care since that day.

—*Coralee Eisner*

CHAPTER 1

Reasons You Should Offer Expanded Dental Services

Introduction

Young men and women spend many long hours and large amounts of money to earn a doctoral degree to learn to care for the animals that share our lives. Most did not attend veterinary school to learn to operate a business. However, the days of graduating, hanging out a shingle, and experiencing success without knowing a great deal about business are over. The veterinarian of today is finding it necessary to take an active role in the management and operation of the practice. Business management is the latest area in which today's owner/veterinarian must become an expert to be successful.

How can a veterinarian succeed in today's market environment? It is necessary to seek new services to target and develop into profitable departments. The goal of this guidebook is to provide you with detailed information about improving the financial performance of your practice by building and marketing a profitable dental department. Along the way, I offer a few golden nuggets that highlight the key points of each section.

Factors That Affect Your Business

A number of factors affect the business aspects of practices today:

▲ **Current market climate and rapidly changing marketplace:** As this guidebook is being written, the economy of the United States is experiencing a period of unparalleled growth, marked by business expansion, high employment, low inflation, and low interest rates. In the last decade, veterinarians have witnessed the growth of pet superstores with veterinary practices, the establishment of corporate practices, and labor shortages. Today, clients are more educated and they are demanding high-quality service and good value for their money.

▲   **Growth of spay/neuter clinics:** In the 1980s, low-cost vaccination clinics sprang up in pet stores, supermarket parking lots, and even the neighboring practice down the street. Spay and neuter clinics offered elective surgery at costs that attracted many pet owners away from full-service practices. The income from these services has been declining rapidly, and many veterinary clinics are finding that they can no longer depend on spay and neuter surgery or vaccinations to provide a significant percentage of production income.

▲   **Potential changes in vaccination protocols:** This is the newest area of controversy in veterinary medicine and it is likely to be years before appropriate protocols are determined. A number of educators, researchers, and veterinary specialty organizations believe that companion animals are being over-vaccinated, and they are lobbying for less frequent vaccinations. Among these groups, the American Board of Feline Practitioners is recommending less frequent vaccination of cats. At the same time, other veterinarians fear the return of the deadly diseases that are so effectively prevented by modern vaccines. While it is still early in the debate, it is clear that seeing a pet less often can result in decreased opportunities to provide the best preventive health care. Certainly, this will have an impact on the bottom line of the unprepared practice.

▲   **Growing competition and the high employment rate:** In the 1990s, large pet superstores have had a major impact on the field of veterinary practice. In February 1998, PETsMART® had 381 superstores in the United States with 188 veterinary clinics employing 370 veterinarians.[1] Initially, traditional practices feared the introduction of the pet superstore, but we are now finding that the veterinary market has expanded to include pet owners who were not previously purchasing veterinary care for their pets. There is a constant demand for new veterinarians to meet the needs of this expanded market. In addition to a shortage of veterinarians, practices are also finding it difficult to fill positions for technicians, receptionists, and hospital assistants with qualified people. The pet superstores offer an attractive package of flexible hours and corporate-sponsored benefits. Well-trained and educated people are asking for and should be paid according to their value as health care team members.

The Importance of the Human–Companion Animal Bond

In the past three decades, the emphasis of pet care has changed. Veterinarians are offering a higher level of care for pets because they have learned that the human–companion animal bond is a significant factor in many people's lives. To many pet owners, their pets are important members of the family. According to an AAHA report, as many as 70 percent of pet owners think of their pets as children. They give their pets human names (51 percent) and pamper them with toys, treats, and premium pet foods. Many are willing to pay higher fees for veterinary care.[2]

People receive different rewards from pet ownership. Single men and women may have pets for companionship, exercise, and as a source of unconditional love. Young married couples may adopt animals as a preliminary experience in parenting. Families may have pets as playmates for their children and as a way to experience the lessons of life and death. Empty nesters and seniors may use pets to reduce the feelings of loneliness and isolation. Pets can provide older citizens with a reason for living. It is well demonstrated that pets can help people live longer and stay healthier. The veterinarian must recognize the importance of the pet to the pet owner and do everything possible to support and promote this bond.[3]

Golden Nugget

Good health care is good business.

Preventive Health Care Is the Key

The companion animal of the 1990s has been the beneficiary of great advances in science, nutrition, technology, and health care. Pet food manufacturers have spent millions of dollars researching nutritional requirements and developing high-quality diets. Vaccines are available that prevent most life-threatening diseases. Safe anesthesia and monitoring, dramatically improved diagnostic services, and high-quality medical care can help pets survive life-threatening illnesses and injuries.

Pet owners want to take good care of their pets. It is up to the veterinarian to educate the client in providing proper pet care. By helping a companion animal to live a long and healthy life, a practice can assure its own financial health. A strong program of preventive health care is the foundation of a successful veterinary practice.

Preventive health care includes:

▲ **Regular physical examinations:** At least once a year, a pet should have a complete physical examination in which every system is carefully evaluated from head to tail. This provides the practitioner with an opportunity to identify problems that the owner may not be aware of and to educate the client in ways to properly care for the pet.

▲ **Appropriate vaccinations:** A young animal requires a strong foundation of vaccinations to protect it against debilitating and deadly diseases. Once an animal is two years old, it should be evaluated annually for risk factors in its lifestyle and be vaccinated appropriately.

▲ **Spay or neuter surgery:** Unless there is a specific reason not to perform the surgery, most pets will benefit from the procedure. The risks of cancer and infection in later years are reduced for both genders. High-risk behaviors that are associated with hormones, such as fence jumping and roaming, are reduced or eliminated.

▲   **Parasite control:** Fecal analysis and heartworm testing are essential to maintain a parasite-free pet in many geographic areas. Parasites should be treated and heartworm preventative prescribed in those locations that are affected by these parasites. Flea and other external parasite control are also important concerns to address in endemic areas.

▲   **Appropriate diagnostic testing to uncover potential health problems:** Laboratory testing and diagnostic imaging are important techniques for uncovering potential diseases that may compromise a pet's health. Initiating a program of routine testing during a pet's middle years can help the veterinarian predict future trends in the pet's long-term health.

▲   **Proper nutrition:** The availability of high-quality, balanced diets designed for life stages has made a big difference in the long-term health of companion animals. Puppies and kittens that are fed high-quality diets can reach their full growth potential. Adult animals, fed the appropriate amount of a diet designed for their life stage, can receive proper nutrition and avoid the problems of obesity. Diets for senior pets help prevent obesity and heart disease and reduce the workload of the kidneys. High-performance diets contribute to optimal conditioning in sporting, working, and service dogs. Prescription diets and specific allergen-free diets are available for pets with special dietary needs. The range of these diets is continually expanding.

▲   **Periodic dental examination and prophylaxis:** It is important to maintain a pet's good oral health because untreated periodontal disease can adversely affect the heart, kidneys, and other organ systems. A pet should have its teeth examined for developmental problems during each vaccination visit as an infant and annually thereafter. The pet with teeth that are showing evidence of plaque, tartar, gingivitis, or oral disease should be scheduled for routine periodic professional dental care and other specific dental care as necessary. As a family member, a pet with halitosis becomes an undesirable companion. By including a program to keep the pet's teeth clean and healthy, the owner can help maintain that pet's role as a family member. It is a win-win situation for the pet, the pet owner, and the veterinarian.

Preventive health care is a program of regularly performed services that, taken as a whole, will help a companion animal live a long and healthy life. This will strengthen and build the human–animal bond, which is the foundation of companion animal practice. With the exception of spay or neuter surgery, each of these components of preventative health care will be performed many times over in a pet's life. Services that you can perform and repeat on a regular basis have the potential to become your profit centers.

Why Is Dentistry Important?

Quality dental care is essential for pets' health for a number of reasons. In addition to the problems associated with periodontal disease itself, animals can develop other systemic disorders.

Periodontal Disease

Periodontal disease is the most common disease in small animal medicine. At the University of Minnesota, in a study of 39,500 dogs, it was found that oral disease was the second most common condition after "healthy" in dogs under 9 years of age.[4] In dogs 10 and older, oral disease was the most common diagnosis. Smaller dogs tend to have more periodontal disease than larger dogs. It is estimated that 80 percent of dogs and 70 percent of cats will show signs of periodontal disease by age three. The lack of dental care can lead to periodontal disease and the loss of teeth. While pet animals can eat without teeth, maintaining the teeth in the mouth improves function for the animal and is more aesthetically pleasing for the owner. Periodontal disease may be painful for an animal and behavior changes have been documented. During acute episodes, pets may experience anorexia, lethargy, fever, and unpredictable behavior. Many pet owners will shun a pet with bad breath. A pet is a better companion when it has clean and healthy teeth. It is much easier and less expensive for an owner to prevent periodontal disease than to treat it or deal with the consequences. As Edward Eisner, DVM, Diplomate AVDC, stated at Veterinary Dentistry '98 in New Orleans, "Teeth—it's like the world—they are worth saving."[5]

Systemic Disease

Dental plaque is a soft sticky substance that begins to form on the surface of the tooth within 3 to 24 hours after tooth cleaning. Plaque is significant because it consists of bacteria, which can lead to gingivitis if not removed. Dental calculus is the hard material formed from plaque and deposited on the teeth. It provides a rough surface for future plaque to adhere to. Plaque can cause gingivitis and lead to eventual bone and tooth loss. It must be removed professionally by the veterinarian under general anesthesia.[6] Left untreated, periodontal disease may lead to systemic disease. The oral cavity serves as a reservoir of bacteria, which can shower the lungs and gain entry to the body. Heart, liver, and kidney disease may result and lead to a shortened life for the pet.[7]

Preventive Dental Care

Regular dental care is important for the long-term health of companion animals. By beginning a program of prevention at an early age, periodontal disease can be avoided. Most people are aware of the frequency of cleanings necessary to maintain their own oral health. Clients depend on their veterinarians to educate them that their pets also need regular cleanings. Most companion animals will benefit from yearly dental cleanings. By being aware of the importance of dentistry, the practitioner can play a significant role in promoting the human–companion animal bond. Performing annual dental examinations and cleanings benefits the pet, the pet owner, and the veterinarian's practice.

Dental Services Are Economical to Offer

After the initial outlay for possible remodeling and necessary dental equipment, most expendable dental supplies are relatively inexpensive. Cleanup following dental procedures is generally quick and does not usually require assembly of sterile packs. Veterinary technicians are trained to perform dental prophylaxis, which can expand the volume of services a practice can provide. This allows the practitioner to do what he or she was trained to do: diagnose, prescribe, and perform surgery.

Dental Services Offer the Opportunity to Develop a Market Niche

A niche is a smaller segment of the market that usually attracts fewer competitors.[8] Veterinary dentistry is an area of expertise that can help you define your practice. With the rapidly changing veterinary marketplace, it is wise to develop skills and services to use to differentiate your practice from other practices in your geographic area. Dental care is a logical niche because nearly all companion animals need periodic dental services.

The Objective of This Guidebook

My goal in this book is to provide you, the practitioner, with a comprehensive guide to starting or expanding a dental department. I first take you through the steps necessary to determine the starting point or baseline against which to measure success. Next, I explain how to develop a marketing plan and set goals. The middle section of the book offers plans for building a dental suite and provides resources for supplies and education. In Chapter 7, I offer marketing ideas and techniques and demonstrate how to implement the marketing plan. In the final sections of the book, I describe how to measure the results of your efforts. Finally, I offer suggestions for fine tuning the marketing plan. You and I are about to embark on an exciting process that will help you and your practice grow.

References

1. L. Brakeman, "Bark Bigger Than Bite," *DVM Newsmagazine* (April 1998): 52.
2. Anonymous, "PR & Marketing Tips: See Sam Run," *AAHA TRENDS Magazine* (April/May 1997): 38–39; Excerpts from AAHA's Sixth Annual Pet Owner Survey (Lakewood, Colo.: AAHA, 1995).
3. R. Hawn, "The Many Faces of Your Clients," *AAHA TRENDS Magazine* (December 1996/January 1997): 7–10.
4. Colin E. Harvey, "Periodontal Disease in Dogs—Etiogenesis, Prevalence, and Significance," in *The Veterinary Clinics of North America, Small Animal Practice, Canine Dentistry* (Philadelphia: W. B. Saunders, 1998): 1123–1124.
5. E. R. Eisner, Personal conversation, at Veterinary Dentistry '98 of the 12th Annual Veterinary Dental Forum, New Orleans, November 1998.
6. Harvey, "Periodontal Disease in Dogs": 1114.
7. L. J. DeBowes, "The Effects of Dental Disease on Systemic Disease," in *The Veterinary Clinics of North America, Small Animal Practice, Canine Dentistry* (Philadelphia: W. B. Saunders, 1998): 1060–1061.
8. P. Kotler, *Marketing Management* (Englewood Cliffs, N.J.: Prentice Hall, Inc., 1991): 264.

CHAPTER 2

The Starting Point

There are two aspects to operating a veterinary practice: how much *income* the practice produces and what *expenses* are associated with producing that income. In this chapter, I show you how to analyze income and expenses to determine the current profitability of your practice. The first step is to understand the concept of the profit center as it is used in this book. Next, I develop a model for determining a starting point so that there is a baseline against which to measure progress.

What Is a Profit Center?

A *profit center* is any set of services that can be provided in such a manner that the income from the services exceeds the associated expenses, leading to a profit or positive net income for the business.

A profit center is sometimes narrowly defined as income from services provided by nonveterinarian sources, such as retail sales, boarding, and grooming. For the purposes of this book, the definition includes services performed by veterinarians and technical staff as well. This broader definition is useful in measuring the performance of veterinarian-provided services. Once income and expense data are collected and analyzed, they can be used to select a clinic department to develop into a profit-producing center through creating and implementing a marketing plan.

The terms *net income* and *profit* are used interchangeably. They both represent how much money is left over after all the bills are paid before the owner is compensated. As the primary investor in the business, the owner should receive a return on the investment in addition to salary. It is the owner's prerogative to determine how much return on investment is desirable and realistic. When creating a budget, it is important to remember to factor in the owner's return on investment as a component of net income. As Robert Froehlich, DVM, MBA, stated, "The bottom line, or net income, is a very deceptive number, since in a small, closely held business, net income [profit] and owners' salaries are virtually interchangeable. Net income must be added to the owners' salaries to get a true picture of profitability."[1] For example, if a practice has an income before owner compensation of $80,000 and the practice owner earns a salary of $70,000, the practice would show a profit of $10,000. The profit would double to $20,000 if the owner was paid a lower salary of $60,000. The owner's salary and net income (profit) will vary. An extreme example of Dr. Froehlich's statement is the owner who simply pays himself or herself what is left over at the end of the month. To properly manage a practice, the business owner should be paid a fair and reasonable salary and set a specific goal to earn a profit, or return on investment, after that salary is paid.

Throughout this book, the profit center model features a hypothetical hospital, the Baseline Animal Hospital. The statistics assigned to the Baseline Animal Hospital are based on a composite distilled from various articles in *TRENDS Magazine*, *Veterinary Economics*, and the *Financial and Productivity Pulsepoints* survey conducted and published by AAHA in 1998. The numbers are meant to serve as an example, not as a benchmark, for comparison with your practice. If an analysis of the income statistics shows that a department is producing a relatively small percentage of income, it is my basic proposition that that particular department has the potential to grow into a profit center.

Using the Profit Center Model

To benefit the most from this section, you need the following information about your practice:

1.   An annual statement of profit and loss from your accounting program or accountant.
2.   The square footage of your facility and your dental department.

Using this information, work through the following steps of the profit center model. Table 2-1 includes the statistics used in the model and the Baseline Animal Hospital, our example.

Table 2-1   Profile of the Baseline Animal Hospital

Gross income/year	$500,000
Staff: Veterinarians	2 full-time
Technicians	2 full-time
Receptionists/Office manager	3 full-time equivalents
Hospital assistants	2 full-time
Square feet of hospital	2,000 sq ft
Hours per week (8–12, 1–6, M–F; 8–1, Sat)	50 hrs
Active clients	2,000
Active animals	3,000
Square feet of dental area	80 sq ft

Table 2-2   Baseline Animal Hospital Income Categories

Department	Income		Percent of Total	
Office visits	$ 50,000	_____	10%	_____
Outpatient treatment	25,000	_____	5	_____
Vaccinations	50,000	_____	10	_____
Pharmacy	80,000	_____	16	_____
Diets and OTC sales	60,000	_____	12	_____
Laboratory	40,000	_____	8	_____
Radiology	15,000	_____	3	_____
Anesthesia	50,000	_____	10	_____
Surgery	25,000	_____	5	_____
Dentistry	10,000	_____	2	_____
Hospitalization	55,000	_____	11	_____
Ancillary services	40,000	_____	8	_____
Total gross income	$500,000	_____	100%	_____

Step 1: Gather Production Income Data

How much production income comes from each department of the hospital? For purposes of simplicity, the income from the Baseline Animal Hospital is divided into 12 income categories. These figures can be found on a monthly income analysis report produced by most veterinary software packages. Income categories can vary widely among practices, reflecting the strengths and interests of each practice. For example, a veterinary dentist might have income categories for each subspecialty of dentistry, such as periodontics or endodontics. Statistics may be compiled manually if no computer is available. Spreadsheet programs are very useful for maintaining summaries of the monthly figures in one worksheet.

In Table 2-2, the income categories of the Baseline Animal Hospital are shown along with the percent of the total income. Following each number is a blank for your personal information. Last year, the Baseline Animal Hospital had a gross production income of $500,000, and income from dental services totaled $10,000, or 2 percent of total income. According to the *Financial and Productivity Pulsepoints* survey conducted by the AAHA, the national average is 1.9 percent for mixed and small animal practices and 2.0 percent for small animal practices only.[2] Let us assume that the owner, Dr. Allright, has recently attended a practice management seminar and believes that his hospital could improve on its dental service package.

Table 2-3   Common Veterinary Expenses

Variable Expenses:	Staff Compensation:
Drugs and medical supplies	Salaries and wages
Diets and pet supplies	Benefit programs
Dental supplies	Medical insurance
Laboratory and radiology	Payroll taxes
Outside laboratory fees	Unemployment taxes
Animal disposal	Workers' compensation insurance
Sales tax	Profit sharing and pensions
	Uniform allowance
Fixed Expenses:	**Associate Veterinarian Compensation:**
Advertising and promotion	Salary
Office and computer supplies	Benefit programs
Postage and printing	Medical insurance
Rent and utilities	Payroll taxes
Insurance	Unemployment taxes
Continuing education	Workers' compensation insurance
Dues, licenses, and subscriptions	Continuing education
Repairs and maintenance	Profit sharing and pensions
Telephone and paging services	
Taxes	**Owner Compensation:**
Charitable donations	Owner salary
Accounting and legal fees	Benefit programs
	Medical insurance
	Owner life and disability insurance
	Profit sharing and pensions
	Payroll taxes
	Unemployment taxes
	Other nondeductible benefits
	Practice vehicle

Source: Adapted from D. L. Tumblin and C. Wutchiett, "Learn to Manage Expenses to Your Advantage," in Veterinary Economics (Lenexa, Kan.: November 1996): 48–55.

Step 2: Prepare Profit and Loss Statement

What is the current financial situation of the Baseline Animal Hospital? The net income of a business is determined by totaling all of the expenses of the business and subtracting the expenses from the total gross income. The hospital's accountant or bookkeeper can provide this report, or an accounting program such as Quickbooks® or PeachTree® can quickly produce the information. Table 2-3 lists some of the most common veterinary expenses.[3] Expenses fall into the following five categories:

1. *Variable expenses* are those that will vary according to the caseload of the hospital. These include expendable supplies, medications, diets, and laboratory and professional fees. The more cases you treat, the greater your expenses will

be. It is helpful to categorize expenses according to the income categories used in Step 1 to facilitate determining the profitability of each department. For example, you can set up a separate account for dental expenses so that they can be compared to dental income.

2. *Fixed expenses* are the general overhead costs of doing business and do not vary significantly with the caseload. Rent, utilities, office supplies, postage, dues, licenses, continuing education, etc., are costs of opening the door. It is money that will be spent no matter how many clients are seen.

3. *Salaries and benefits for staff members.* Components of this category are listed in Table 2-3. For the profit and loss statement, staff salaries are considered fixed expenses and vary little with caseload.

4. *Salaries and benefits for associate veterinarians.* Salaries and benefits for associate veterinarians are excluded from fixed expenses because they are often based on a percent of the associates' production income and could vary substantially. It is also helpful to monitor the percentages of "profit before veterinarian compensation" and "associate compensation" for practice management purposes.

5. *Salaries and benefits for the practice owner(s).* This catagory includes all compensation that the owners pay themselves. It should include all espenses paid for by the practice that specifically benefit the owners.

Table 2-4 shows the profit and loss statement for the example hospital. The Baseline Animal Hospital has a fairly typical income picture. Dr. Allright has a slightly better than average salary and benefit income and a small amount of net income left over. By focusing on building a dental department, he is hoping that he can improve his bottom line.

Step 3: Calculate Overhead of Hospital

The Baseline Animal Hospital's profit and loss statement in Table 2-4 is displayed in the form of a management statement. The management statement is useful because it is organized to reveal a realistic estimation of net income. Each of the five expense categories is listed in order. The variable expenses in the example total $120,000 and fixed expenses total $115,000. After adding staff salaries and benefits ($115,000), the total expenses are $360,000 or 72 percent of gross income. This leaves the practice $140,000 to pay the associate veterinarian and the owner and show a small profit.

To calculate the hospital overhead per square foot, fixed expenses ($115,000) and nonveterinarian staff wages ($115,000) are added and the sum ($230,000) is divided by the square footage (2,000 square feet). Staff salaries are included as fixed expenses because they are expenses that will be incurred whatever the workload. In the example, the fixed overhead per square foot is $115. The next figure to derive is the cost per minute of opening the doors every business day. The Baseline Animal Hospital is open 50 hours per week for 52 weeks a year, less one week for holidays. This calculates to 153,000 minutes per year. By dividing the total annual overhead

Table 2-4   Baseline Animal Hospital Statement of Profit and Loss

Account	(Expense)	Income	Percent of Total Income
Gross income		$500,000	100%
Variable expenses			
Medicines	(50,000)		10
Clinic supplies	(25,000)		5
Diets and OTC	(25,000)		5
Dental supplies	**(500)**		**.1**
Lab, surgery, X-ray	(10,000)		2
Outside lab fees	(9,500)		1.9
Subtotal	*(120,000)*		*24*
Outside professional services	(10,000)		2
Total Variable Expenses	*(130,000)*		*26*
Fixed expenses			
Office supplies and equipment	(25,000)		5
Housing expense	(60,000)		12
Other deductible expenses	(30,000)		6
Total Fixed Expenses	*(115,000)*		*23*
Salaries and wages (support staff only)	(115,000)		23
Total Fixed Expenses and Staff Salaries and Wages	*(230,000)*		*46*
TOTAL EXPENSES	**(360,000)**		72
Profit before veterinarian compensation		**140,000**	28
Less salary and benefits for associate DVM	(50,000)		10
Cash available to owner		**90,000**	18
Less depreciation expense	(10,000)		2
Less owner's salary and benefits	(70,000)		14
NET INCOME		**10,000**	2
Total fixed expenses and staff salaries and wages/2,000 sq ft	$ 115.00/sq ft		

Table 2-5   Cost per Minute of Doing Business

Fixed expenses	$115,000
Staff salaries and benefits	115,000
Total overhead	$230,000
Divided by minutes open per year	153,000
Equals cost per minute	$1.50

Table 2-6   Dental Department Profitability

Statistic	Amount
Number of dental cases	200
Average fee	$50
Income from dentistry	$10,000
Space for dental department	80 sq ft
Overhead/sq ft	$115
Overhead charged to dentistry	$9,200
Direct dental expenses	$500
Total dental department expense	$9,700
Net dental income before veterinarian compensation	$300

by the minutes open per year, we have determined that the cost per minute of doing business is $1.50, as illustrated in Table 2-5. This will be useful information for setting dental fees, as discussed in Chapter 6.

Step 4: Calculate the Profitability of the Dental Department
With the information we have gathered, it is now possible to calculate the current profitability of the dental department at the Baseline Animal Hospital. As we demonstrated for the hospital as a whole, the same procedure applies to individual departments. The hospital produced $10,000 in dental income (see Table 2-2) against $500 for dental expenses (see Table 2-4), showing an apparent profit of $9,500. This does not, however, include the wages earned by a veterinary technician while cleaning the teeth, the rent, electricity, telephone, and other expenses involved with scheduling the appointment and admitting the patient. To obtain a true picture of dental department profitability, it is necessary to assign a share of the overhead expense. To allocate overhead costs to the dental department, multiply the overhead per square foot times the square footage that the dental department occupies. Professional income from dental services minus direct costs of dental supplies and overhead allocated to the department equals the profit or loss from the dental department, as illustrated in Table 2-6. We see that the dental department is contributing $300 to the profit before veterinarian compensation.

If there is no separate dental area, it will be necessary to allocate some square footage to create a baseline. To estimate how much room you will need, multiply the square footage of the treatment room by the percent of income derived from delivering dental care compared to the total income produced in the treatment room. For example, the treatment room in Hospital XYZ is 20 feet by 15 feet or 300 square feet and the room is used for minor surgery, treatments, and radiology as well as dentistry. If dental income is 25 percent of the income produced in the treatment room, we can allocate 25 percent of the 300 square feet, or 75 square feet, to dentistry's share of the overhead.

Table 2-7   Baseline Animal Hospital Combined Dental and Anesthesia Income and Expenses

	Dental Income/Expenses	Anesthesia Income/Expenses From Dentistry	Combined Income/Expenses
Income	$10,000	$10,000 (20% of cases)	$20,000
Direct expenses	500	2,000 (200 cases x $10/case)	2,500
Overhead	9,200	4,600 ($115 x 40 sq ft)	13,800
Total expenses	$9,700	$6,600	$16,300
Net dental income before veterinarian compensation	$300	$3,400	$3,700

It is also possible to assign a portion of anesthesia income to obtain a more accurate picture of the income the dental department is producing. Because dental procedures are normally performed under general anesthesia, combining the two categories will yield a more accurate baseline to measure against. Because anesthesia income is produced at the same time as dental income, the allocation can be somewhat arbitrary, but it is possible to make a close estimate.

Assume the following about the Baseline Animal Hospital. Anesthesia income is produced primarily by the surgery, radiology, and dental departments; the "procedure" income from these four categories (anesthesia, surgery, radiology, and dentistry) totals 20 percent of the total hospital income. Add 20 percent of the anesthesia income to dental income, because dentistry is 20 percent of the radiology, surgery, and dentistry combined. Assume that these three departments occupy 20 percent of the clinic space or 400 square feet. Since dental income is 10 percent of the total procedure income ($10,000 ÷ [$15,000 + $50,000 + $25,000 + $10,000]), allocate 10 percent of this room or 40 square feet for anesthesia overhead expense as applied to the dental caseload. When this process is completed, it is determined that the dental department has contributed $3,700 to profit before veterinarian compensation (see Table 2-7). After the Baseline Animal Hospital develops a marketing plan for dentistry (see Chapter 8), it will be possible to demonstrate how these results may be improved.

References

1. R. Froehlich, "The Health of Your Practice—Understanding Financial Profiles," *AAHA TRENDS Magazine* (April/May 1992): 23–25.
2. E. Bohlender, *Financial and Productivity Pulsepoints* (Lakewood, Colo.: AAHA Press, 1998): 18.
3. D. L. Tumblin and C. Wutchiett, "Learn to Manage Expenses to Your Advantage," *Veterinary Economics* (November 1996): 48–55.

CHAPTER 3

Create a Marketing Plan

Wouldn't it be nice if it were enough to simply decide to "do more dentistry"? At a basic level, a practitioner could begin by performing an oral examination on every patient and scheduling a dental cleaning for each one that showed tartar on its teeth. If the doctors at the Baseline Animal Hospital performed 10 percent more dental cleanings at the same fee, they could increase their production income by $1,000, of which approximately $950 would become net income. While this might appear to be a successful approach, it is a hit-or-miss procedure that may lead to uncertain results. The purpose of this chapter and this guidebook is to go beyond the "quick fix" and to offer the tools to make a difference in the level of service that the practice is providing its clientele and patients. While the basic goal is to "do more dentistry," the ability to "do better dentistry" will carry a practice beyond the entry level. To achieve this goal your practice needs a marketing plan.

Developing a marketing plan can be fairly straightforward. The process is to develop a mission, set goals, identify areas that can be targeted for improvement, and create some steps to implement the plan. Philip Kotler has defined strategic planning in *Marketing Management*.

> Strategic planning is the managerial process of developing and maintaining a viable fit between the organization's objectives and resources and its changing market opportunities. The aim of strategic planning is to shape and reshape the company's business and products so that they combine to produce satisfactory profits and growth.[1]

This chapter outlines a step-by-step process for creating a marketing plan for the Baseline Animal Hospital. The completed plan appears in Appendix A.

Step 1: Develop a Mission and Goals

The first step is to develop a mission relating to dental care. A mission is a broad statement that describes in general terms the type of dental care the practice wants to offer. The assumption of this guidebook is that your primary financial mission is to develop a profitable dental department. From the perspective of the human–animal bond, the mission is to provide better dental services to the pets entrusted to our care so that they can continue to contribute to the lives of their owners by experiencing good health. It is important to remember to put the needs of the patient and client first. If a client senses that the veterinarian is motivated primarily by money, he or she may be turned off to the practice. Good health care and good business are compatible. Providing high-quality medical care in a well-managed practice environment will result in growth of the business. A practice may offer several levels of dental services:

▲ **Basic dental care:** These services should be offered at every veterinary hospital. Basic dental cleaning includes ultrasonic scaling, subgingival curettage, and polishing, all with the patient under general anesthesia.

▲ **Intermediate level dentistry:** Most animals will experience fractured teeth and/or periodontal disease during their lives. Repairing the injured tooth, rather than extracting it, is less painful for the patient and allows the continued use of the tooth. Practices that perform this service can charge higher fees because the service is less commonly offered. Most animals experience periodontal disease during their lives, and in-hospital treatment and home care training can be added to the services offered. Periodontal disease is so prevalent that the service should be offered in-house rather than referring the patient to a specialist.

▲ **Advanced specialized veterinary dentistry:** Periodontics, endodontics, orthodontics, restorative dentistry, and dental surgery are advanced level dentistry. Veterinarians who can perform advanced dental procedures are offering a service that has great value to many people to whom their pets' welfare is paramount. These clients are proud of providing the best care and quality of life for their four-legged family members. They are willing to pay premium prices for the best care possible. Advanced dental care can contribute dramatically to the bottom line of a practice.

It takes two to six years of study to become a specialist in veterinary dentistry, but intermediate levels of competence are not difficult to achieve. After reading through the steps for the market analysis, you will need to determine which level of dentistry you want to deliver. The setting of a mission is a fluid process and the result is rarely carved in stone. Once the first level of care is achieved, you may be either satisfied with the results or encouraged to advance beyond your initial success. This guidebook offers information and resources to help you set up a dental practice beginning at the basic level and advancing to higher levels.

Once your mission has been determined, you can develop more specific goals. According to Tom Loebach, marketing director, AAHA, "A goal can be thought of as a statement that contributes to the mission of the hospital. It tends to be abstract, inspirational, and visionary."[2] An example of a goal could be "We will improve the quality of the dental care delivered at our hospital." Dr. Allright and his staff adopted this goal and developed four additional goals for their marketing plan:

1. **Patient care:** We will improve the quality of the dental care delivered at our hospital.

2. **Finance:** We will increase the volume of dental care provided to improve our financial position.

3. **Facility and equipment:** We will expand the dental department of this hospital by purchasing the best equipment that we can afford to provide higher quality dental services.

4. **Education:** Our doctors and staff members will become more knowledgeable about dental health through continuing education courses and reading. We will encourage our staff to grow and develop to each individual's potential.

5. **Marketing:** We will develop marketing tools to increase client awareness of dental health.

Step 2: Perform a Market Analysis

Before making the great leap into offering veterinary dentistry, it is helpful and necessary to examine your local market. The more you know about your hospital, your competition, and the business environment in your area, the better you will be able to develop a set of services that your clients will find desirable and be willing to purchase. Performing a market analysis will help you learn about your current situation and illuminate areas for improvement. It is also very useful to survey your clients and ask them how they value the attributes and services of your practice. The process will help you find your starting point and begin to map out a plan of action. To learn more about your situation, this section analyzes internal and external business environments.

We will perform a SWOT analysis, in which we look at the practice's internal strengths and weaknesses, and the external opportunities and threats that confront it. This is a process of asking questions, and the answers should tell you where to focus your efforts to improve your dental practice. It lends itself well to staff involvement and is great subject material for staff meetings. The more your staff participates in the market analysis and goal setting, the easier it will be to gain their cooperation in building a dental practice.[3]

The SWOT analysis begins with a discussion of the external environment (opportunities and threats). By first analyzing the competitive environment and listing the external forces acting on the hospital, it is easier to focus on the internal strengths and weaknesses and gain a more useful understanding of the local veterinary market.

External Environment Analysis (Opportunities and Threats)

The first step is to list the factors in the external environment that could have an impact on the ability of the hospital to be competitive. These are generally forces beyond the control of the practice. Some of these factors are listed in Table 3-1. If a statement is relevant to your situation, check it off. The lists are not intended to be all-inclusive; you may wish to list other situations that may have an impact on your practice. A marketing *opportunity* is an attractive area for a marketing program in which the hospital could enjoy a competitive advantage. A *threat* is a challenge presented by an unfavorable trend or development that could lead to erosion of the hospital's position in the absence of a purposeful marketing action.[4] Be aware that some threats may also serve as opportunities and the reverse may be true as well.

Table 3-1   External Environment Checklist

✓	Opportunities	✓	Threats
☐	The local economy is growing. Employment is high.	☐	The local economy is shrinking and in a recession.
☐	New businesses are coming into the area offering jobs.	☐	Businesses are leaving the area. Unemployment is high.
☐	The practice is located in a good location: lots of potential traffic.	☐	The practice location is poor. There is a high vacancy rate in the nearby stores.
☐	There is no nearby veterinary competition.	☐	There are a number of veterinary practices located nearby.
☐	Opportunity to specialize: There are no veterinary dentists in the area.	☐	Threat of competition: There is a veterinary dentist within the area.
☐	The pet superstore is far from your practice.	☐	A pet superstore is nearby and offers discount services.
☐	This is an urban practice: high density of pet owners.	☐	The practice is in a rural area. Pet owners tend to use home remedies.
☐	The clientele can afford high-quality pet care.	☐	The clientele can't afford high-quality care for pets.
☐	The area has a high standard of veterinary care and clients expect it.	☐	The standard of veterinary care in the area is average. Clients are money conscious.
☐	The practice offers easy access and plentiful parking.	☐	Access to the practice is difficult and parking is limited.
☐	There is an opportunity to expand facilities, if necessary.	☐	Your landlord wants to redevelop your property, and you may have to move.
☐	The local veterinary association works with the animal shelters to promote local practices.	☐	Local shelters offer spay/neuter services, creating a more competitive environment.

According to Edward Eisner, DVM, Diplomate of the AVDC, of the Denver Veterinary Dental Service, "There is enough dental pathology that, if a practice were serving its patients well, a solo practitioner could hire a full-time veterinarian and a full-time technician to perform only the dentistry in that practice." Even if there is a dental specialist in your area, there are more than enough dental opportunities in your own practice if you are interested in elevating your level of dental care.

Internal Environment Analysis (Strengths and Weaknesses)
The second step of the market analysis is to examine carefully the strengths and weaknesses of your hospital. Take a close look at your facility and equipment, client base, staff members, training levels of all employees, and any other factors that you feel might have an impact on the dental mission. Listed in Table 3-2 are factors to consider when evaluating your strengths and weaknesses. The form allows you to rate each as a major strength, minor strength, neutral, minor weakness, or major weakness. Grading the various factors will help you visualize your current position and begin the process of capitalizing on your strengths and correcting your weaknesses. Some factors will be more important to you than others, and the last column allows you to rate each item.

Table 3-2   Internal Environment Analysis

Factor	Performance					Importance		
	Major Strength	Minor Strength	Neutral	Minor Weakness	Major Weakness	Hi	Med	Low
Physical facilities	___	___	___	___	___	—	—	—
Dental equipment	___	___	___	___	___	—	—	—
Capacity	___	___	___	___	___	—	—	—
Office hours	___	___	___	___	___	—	—	—
Profitability	___	___	___	___	___	—	—	—
Availability of capital	___	___	___	___	___	—	—	—
Financial stability	___	___	___	___	___	—	—	—
Dedicated staff	___	___	___	___	___	—	—	—
Staff training/ technical skill	___	___	___	___	___	—	—	—
Veterinarian training and interest	___	___	___	___	___	—	—	—
Hospital reputation	___	___	___	___	___	—	—	—
Marketing program	___	___	___	___	___	—	—	—
Visionary leadership	___	___	___	___	___	—	—	—
Client base	___	___	___	___	___	—	—	—
Computer system	___	___	___	___	___	—	—	—

Table 3-3   Performance-Importance Matrix

	Low Performance	High Performance
High Importance	A. Concentrate here	B. Keep up the good work
Low Importance	C. Low priority	D. Possible to overdo it here

After rating these factors, combine the performance and importance ratings for four possible results, as illustrated in the matrix in Table 3-3. For any hospital, items that fall in cell A are important and require improvement. If a hospital is doing well on items in cell B, successful efforts should be continued. In cell C are less important factors, which will need improvement at a later time. Finally, in cell D are unimportant factors that are rated as strengths.[5] It would be appropriate to put energy and resources in weaker areas. For example, the Baseline Animal Hospital employs two technicians who enjoy cleaning teeth. This important strength will be instrumental in building the dental department and the technicians' interest should be encouraged. On the other hand, the ultrasonic cleaner is broken and the lack of dental equipment is a major weakness. It is difficult to build a department when you have trouble performing the service. Dr. Allright can see quickly that it would be best to focus on repairing or replacing his dental equipment so that his strengths, the technicians, can "keep up the good work." Improving the dental department will support and improve staff morale and will also assist practice growth.

Table 3-4 shows the results of the SWOT analysis done for our example, Baseline Animal Hospital.

Step 3: Establish Objectives

After defining the mission and completing the SWOT analysis, you can more clearly visualize your current position. You should have found both strengths and opportunities on which to capitalize and weaknesses and threats that need to be remedied. The next step is to set goals and objectives.

Objectives can include increasing numbers of dental examinations and cleanings, remedying the weaknesses discovered in the SWOT analysis, educating your clientele about the importance of dental care, improving marketing effectiveness, or purchasing/leasing equipment. Specific numerical objectives are useful for comparison against a baseline and make it easier to quantify the results. Examples could be to increase dental cleanings by 25 percent or increase dental income by 10 percent. Stephen Fisher, DVM, vice president of business development and recruiting for Veterinary Centers of America, suggests a benchmark of 15 to 30 dental procedures per veterinarian per month.[6] If Dr. Allright decided to use this benchmark, he could set a goal of increasing the average number of dental procedures per veterinarian from the

Table 3-4   Results of the SWOT Analysis for the Baseline Animal Hospital

Strengths	Weaknesses
Good reputation in the community	Ultrasonic scaler broken
Strong interest in dentistry	Lack of dental expertise
Well-trained, motivated staff	Lack of dental equipment
Adequate facility, room to grow	Clientele uninformed about dental care
Newsletter	Limited budget
Up-to-date computer system	Profitability marginal, limited funds to
Some marketing experience	develop dentistry
No outstanding loans	
Opportunities	**Threats**
Local economy strong	Local competition is strong
Hospital is in a good location with good visibility	Pet superstore within three miles, and it has a
Dental specialist in neighboring city	full-service hospital
Good standard of veterinary care in the	Local geographic area is stable, little
community	opportunity for growth in client numbers
Clients are willing to pay above-average fees	

current 8.3 to 15 per month. The range of objectives is unlimited and the results of SWOT analysis are a good place to start when setting this range. The key is to develop the objectives based on the amount of time the practice owner and the staff are willing to put into this effort and the amount of resources you need to succeed.[7] It is better to be conservative and achieve the desired results than to aim for more than you can accomplish and become discouraged by failure. In other words, set objectives that are reasonably achievable so that you *can* succeed. Success builds on success.

Using the Baseline Animal Hospital as an example, after performing the SWOT analysis, Dr. Allright learned that his greatest strengths were his desire to learn, the positive attitude of his staff, and the other existing features of his practice that could be used to grow and expand his services: his reputation, computer system, and marketing experience. His weaknesses are his existing dental equipment and limited financial resources. His hospital experiences strong local competition, and Dr. Allright feels that the opportunity to develop a dental niche is very attractive. He is friendly with the specialist in the neighboring city and may be able to observe him practicing advanced level dentistry. With this in mind, Dr. Allright and his staff develop a set of objectives at a staff meeting:

1. Educate the clientele about the importance of dental care.
2. Provide above-average dental services, beginning with dental prophylaxis.
3. Perform a dental examination during every physical examination, whether the patient is healthy or ill.
4. Schedule animals that have tartar buildup or inflamed gums for dental cleanings.

5. Double the production volume for dental services in each of the next two years. This will increase dental income to 8 percent of total production.

6. Consider expanding dental services to endodontics and periodontics once basic services are well established.

7. Budget $5,000 for continuing education, repairs, and purchases of dental equipment in each of the next two years. A dental X-ray machine (approximately $3,000) and a new, moderately priced dental delivery system ($2,000–3,000) are at the top of the capital equipment wish list.

Step 4: Create Strategies

Creating a strategic marketing plan involves using your imagination to envision the results of your labors. What is your "vision of success"?[8] Where do you see your practice in one, three, and five years with respect to your dental services? Can you imagine a practice with happy clients whose pets live in good health to beyond normal life expectancies? Are your clients so pleased with your services that they refer their friends, relatives, and neighbors to you? What does success look like in your dream? What strategies will be used to implement the objectives established in Step 3? How will the services be marketed internally and externally? A strategy is a plan of action or policy to achieve your "vision of success." They are the broad steps to get from where you are now to where you want to be in the next three to five years. The next chapters offer the tools and information to achieve your objectives. Dr. Allright and his staff developed a list of strategies to accomplish their objectives (see Table 3-5). In the righthand column is space for you to fill in your strategies.

Step 5: Develop an Action Plan

The action plan is the detailed plan for the implementation of the strategies outlined in the last step. These are concrete actions that describe who, what, when, where, why, and how for each step. An action plan for the Baseline Animal Hospital is shown in Appendix A. An action plan should specify the following:

▲ *Who* will be responsible for the action? Will the veterinarian, a technician, a receptionist, or an outside source perform this action?

▲ *What* is the specific action and which strategy does it address?

▲ *When* is this action to be completed? Develop a timeline for the strategy.

▲ *Where* will this action take place? Will this be performed in the office or elsewhere?

▲ *Why* is this action necessary? There should be a specific reason for each action to be performed.

▲ *How* will this action be implemented? What techniques will be used?

▲ *How* will the results be measured? Can they be quantified so that the degree of success can be evaluated?[9]

Table 3-5   Marketing Strategies

Baseline Animal Hospital Strategies	Your Strategies
1. Continuing education: find basic level dental courses in local area for veterinarians and staff members.	_____
2. Repair existing dental equipment.	_____
3. Purchase equipment for basic level dentistry.	_____
4. Produce newsletter focused on dental care.	_____
5. Educate clients about dental care during examination visits.	_____
6. Use reminders for dental recalls.	_____
7. Begin photographing dental cases for client education. Make a "Smile Book."	_____

Step 6: Monitor Results

After the action plan is implemented, it is important to monitor the results to measure your success. If the results of the marketing plan fall short of your desired goal, analyze the reasons and institute changes. The process of monitoring the results is discussed in more detail in Chapter 8. Creating and implementing a marketing plan is an ongoing repetitive process of setting goals, developing an action plan, implementing the plan, and monitoring the results. After each sequence, fine-tune the action plan to improve the results. There will be times when you may want to re-evaluate your goals and adjust them to reflect a new reality; for example, a goal might be achieved easily and you might wish to raise the target level. By going through this process, you will be able to elevate the level of dentistry practiced in your hospital and eventually achieve your vision of success.

References

1. P. Kotler, *Marketing Management* (Englewood Cliffs, N.J.: Prentice Hall, Inc., 1988): 33.
2. T. Loebach, "A Simplified Approach to Strategic Planning," *AAHA TRENDS Magazine* (October/November 1990): 33.
3. Ibid.: 34.
4. Kotler, *Marketing Management:* 48–49.
5. Ibid.: 50–52.
6. S. C. Fisher, "Associates in Practice: Production Reports Provide Great Feedback," *DVM Newsmagazine* (December 1998): 46.
7. J. B. McCarthy, *Basic Guide to Veterinary Hospital Management* (Lakewood, Colo.: AAHA Press, 1995): 88–89.
8. Loebach, "Simplified Approach to Strategic Planning": 34.
9. G. L. Jordan and M. Sheahan, "Should You Strategically Manage Your Practice?" *AAHA TRENDS Magazine* (October/November 1997): 12.

CHAPTER 4

Education and Enlightenment

Golden Nugget

Dental education is contagious.
The more you learn about it, the more excited you get.
—Dr. Debra Fiorito, Diplomate AVDC[1]

At the most basic level, a practitioner can decide to increase the number of dental cleanings by simply deciding to do just that. However, the purpose of this guide-book is to help you improve not just the quantity but also the *quality* of dental services. To promote expanded services in the dental profit center, it is essential to have the knowledge and experience to provide the target service at a level that is at or above the level of accepted care in your community. You will need to take the lead in gaining the education and experience to proceed with the development of the dental department. You will most likely be the individual responsible for training and educating the staff in the benefits and techniques of offering dental services.

Dental Education

Once the scope of the services is decided, you will need to determine how much education you require to gain the expertise and experience you need to offer your services at a competent level. Courses are widely offered at continuing education seminars in the United States and around the world. For the most current information, consult the listings in the back pages of the *AAHA TRENDS Magazine* and the *Journal of the American Veterinary Medical Association,* as well as state and local associations. In addition to seminars, there are an increasing number of reference books on the subject of veterinary dentistry and Internet web sites devoted to veterinary dentistry. Courses are offered at entry level, intermediate, and advanced levels to accommodate the needs of all practitioners. Following are lists of associations and resources that offer dental education.

National Veterinary Associations
> American Animal Hospital Association
> 12575 West Bayaud Ave.
> Lakewood, CO 80228
> Member Service Center Telephone: 800-883-6301
> *www.healthypet.com*
> The AAHA offers national and regional meetings and publications.

> American Veterinary Medical Association
> 1931 North Meacham Rd., Suite 100
> Schaumburg, IL 60173-4360
> Telephone: 800-248-2862
> The AVMA offers an annual national meeting and publications.

Dental Specialty Associations in the United States
The dental specialty groups present an annual dental forum every fall that offers the most comprehensive range of veterinary dental courses available today. The conference offers more than 150 seminars and wet laboratories for all levels of expertise and an exhibit hall for dental equipment and supplies. For information about the three groups discussed below and the annual dental forum, contact:

> Veterinary Dental Associations Office
> 530 Church St., Suite 700
> Nashville, TN 37210
> Telephone: 800-332-AVDS (2837)
> Fax: 615-254-7047
> e-mail: dgreen@wmgt.org

The quarterly *Journal of Veterinary Dentistry,* published by the American Veterinary Dental Society, is the official journal of the following three groups.

▲ **American Veterinary Dental Society (AVDS):** The AVDS is for all who are interested in veterinary dentistry. The society includes veterinarians, veterinary technicians, dentists, and corporations who wish to be informed about meetings, groups, and the latest developments in veterinary dentistry.

▲ **Academy of Veterinary Dentistry (AVD):** The AVD is for those with an elevated interest in veterinary dentistry. Membership is not limited to veterinarians. The members become Fellows of the AVD through a process of submitting credentials and sitting for an examination.

▲ **American Veterinary Dental College (AVDC):** The AVDC is the official AVMA specialty dental organization for veterinarians only. Members become diplomates in veterinary dentistry through a rigorous process of extensive training, building a credential package, and an examination. The AVDC updates the annual meeting web site at *www://ourworld.compuserve.com/homepages/texasvet1.*

International Veterinary Associations

Veterinary associations around the world offer dental courses, and there are dental specialty groups in Europe, Great Britain, Japan, and Australia. The annual World Veterinary Dental Congress is frequently held in conjunction with the World Small Animal Veterinary Association (WSAVA) meeting. The Veterinary Dental Congress attracts veterinarians worldwide and offers all levels of seminars and laboratories on veterinary dentistry. Recently the European Veterinary Dental College was founded; it is comparable to the AVDC in requirements and testing.

> World Small Animal Veterinary Association
> David Wadsworth
> c/o British Small Animal Veterinary Association
> Kingsley House
> Church Lane, Shurdington
> Chettenham, Gloucestershire GL SISTQ
> United Kingdom
> Telephone: 011-44-1242-862994
> Fax: 011-44-1242-863009
> e-mail: david@wadders.demon.co.uk

The contact address for the WSAVA follows the office of the secretary. This is the September 1999 address. It is also possible to contact the office of the executive director of the AAHA for current information about the WSAVA.

Other Continuing Education Opportunities

1. **State and local meetings:** Consult your local veterinary associations for information about dental programs. These groups also appreciate input for their continuing education topics, and many of the diplomates of the AVDC are available for speaking engagements.

2. **Seminars sponsored by corporations that service the veterinary industry:** Pharmacia and Upjohn, IDEXX, Periogene, and Virbac are a few companies that offer seminars at various locations around the United States.

3. **University courses/veterinary schools:** Veterinary schools sometimes offer short courses in dental topics. The schools that have a resident dental specialist are likely to offer more comprehensive programs.

Local Veterinary Dental Specialists

Many dental specialists are willing to train their colleagues in dental techniques. There are mentoring programs for practitioners who are interested in advanced training leading to becoming a specialist. Some specialists are also willing to train technicians in techniques of oral examination and dental prophylaxis.

Local Dentists

Dentists in your local area are some of the best sources for information on local availability of dental equipment, supplies, and repairs. Many dentists are interested in veterinary dentistry because it offers something new and out of the ordinary for them, and they are happy to be of service.

Books and Periodicals

There are increasing numbers of reference books devoted to veterinary dentistry. These books are updated regularly to include recent advancements in scientific research and techniques. The 1999 suggested reading list for the candidates for diplomate of the AVDC is included in Appendix B.

Videotapes and CD-ROMs

Videotapes that can be used as training aids, when attending a continuing education meeting is not practical, are available from various sources. Several videotape series, produced by veterinary dentists, are available, as well as tapes produced by manufacturers that explain how to use their products. Examples of such tapes are VRx, Oral Examination Training Kit; Denmat's Video Series; Engler, Practical Veterinary Dentistry; and Periogene, Ultrasonic Scaling Technique.

Web Sites

The following web sites are monitored by the AVDC:

▲ NOAH (AVMA) site: www.avma.org/network.html

▲ VIN site: www.mother.com/~vin/

Golden Nugget

Veterinary hospitals that use their support staff to the fullest find that their doctor's personal gross revenues increase dramatically, as does hospital profitability.

—Jeff Rothstein, DVM, MBA[2]

Staff Training: A Stepping Stone to Success

A well-trained support staff of veterinary technicians and front office personnel is essential to creating a profitable dental center. Offering premium dental services to your clientele requires the cooperation of the entire team. A staff member who is undereducated about the importance of high-quality dental care will lack the knowledge to communicate this to your clients. It pays to delegate as much as possible to the support staff as long as they are capable and qualified to perform the task.[3] By educating the staff, they in turn will be able to adequately promote veterinary dentistry. There are continuing education courses available for technicians at the national meetings, but often it is the practitioner's responsibility to train the staff members in the value and procedures of veterinary dentistry.

Front Office Staff

The reception staff should be knowledgeable about the process and benefits of periodic dental care and be able to explain and promote the services and dental products to your clientele. The importance of receptionists cannot be overstated, because they are usually the first and the last people that your client will have contact with during a visit.

Veterinary Technicians

The technicians are key team members who can perform an essential and valuable role in veterinary dentistry. In most cases, trained veterinary technicians can perform the majority of the dental prophylaxes and assist in advanced dental techniques. Because technicians are paid on a lower scale than veterinarians, the more the practitioner can delegate to technicians, the more profitable the department will be. It is highly cost effective to develop a well-trained dental team that can increase the volume of professional services performed at your facility. Technicians' skills and duties may include the following:

1. Explaining treatment plans and educating clients about dental care and procedures.
2. Charting oral pathology and updating patient dental records.
3. Taking oral radiographs.
4. Performing dental prophylaxis quickly, thoroughly, and efficiently.
5. Identifying dental problems that may require advanced level dental therapy and alerting the practitioner. This can be a major practice builder for those hospitals that offer advanced level dental care.
6. Becoming valuable chairside assistants for advanced dental procedures. This can improve clinic efficiency and increase production income.
7. Performing the maintenance and cleaning of dental equipment and handpieces.
8. Maintaining the dental operatory and a well-stocked inventory of dental supplies.
9. Delivering discharge instructions and teaching home care to clients.[4]

Training for Veterinary Technicians

The formal training that veterinary technicians receive in dental prophylaxis during their initial studies will be basic, and practical experience will be limited. Veterinarians or other technicians on the staff will train most new technicians on the job. Continuing education opportunities for staff members are often offered in conjunction with programs for veterinarians, but they are generally on a basic level. Many of the national meetings and state and local associations will offer dental topics and technicians are often welcome at the programs that are given for veterinarians. In addition, state technician associations and the veterinary technician schools may offer dental courses as well. The topics relevant for technicians would cover the duties previously listed.

The American Society of Veterinary Dental Technicians (ASVDT) is an association dedicated to veterinary dentistry. The ASVDT is a society for veterinary technicians and assistants and dental hygienists interested in veterinary dentistry. The AVDS's *Journal of Veterinary Dentistry* is also the official journal of the ASVDT. The ASVDT holds a national annual technician meeting in conjunction with the Veterinary Dental Forum and publishes a periodic newsletter containing educational articles and information about the society and its activities. The ASVDT also offers a home study course and first-level qualifying examination that includes two teaching videos, a video-related workbook, a reference compendium, and an examination, for $75 for members. After passing the examination, the member receives a certificate designating him or her as qualified in veterinary dental health. Contact the ASVDT at:

> American Society of Veterinary Dental Technicians
> P.O. Box 1636
> Venice, FL 34284-1636
> Telephone: 800-613-3647; 941-488-7802
> Fax: 941-484-1439

References

1. C. Chapman, "Let The Dental Prophy Polish Your Bottom Line," *Veterinary Economics* (February 1996): 75.
2. J. Rothstein, "Staff Leveraging Grows Talents, Profits," *Veterinary Product News* (April 1998): 26–27.
3. Ibid.
4. Jan Bellows, DVM, "Working With Your Dental Team," *Conference Proceedings of the 11th Annual Veterinary Dental Forum of the American Veterinary Dental College,* Denver, Colorado, 1997: 275–279.

CHAPTER 5

Designing and Equipping Your Dental Suite

When designing your dental suite, your budget and the space available for a dental department will limit your decisions. In 1992, the Floyd Dental Suite opened at the University of California–Davis at a cost of $200,000. This state-of-the-art dental suite featured cantilevered workstations with contoured Corian countertops; fold-away, under-the-counter dental delivery systems; rolling dental carts; wall-mounted anesthesia delivery systems; and foldaway X-ray and lighting. Depending on your financial situation, you can incorporate many of these features when you design your dental facility.[1]

If you have the luxury of allocating a separate room for a dental suite (anything bigger than an unused closet), your options will be much broader. An unlimited budget and an extra room would be ideal. Because most of us live in the real world and lack these choices, this chapter offers ideas for dental departments that can be integrated into a treatment room as well as for a dedicated dental suite. If you plan to add dental equipment to an existing treatment area, you may already have some features in place, such as a tub table with plumbing. When researching this chapter, I asked a number of diplomates of the American Veterinary Dental College what features they liked and disliked about their dental operatories and what advice they would like to offer. Their responses and suggestions are presented in the following Golden Nugget. One of your best resources is an architect or space planner, especially one who has experience in veterinary hospital design. An extensive list of suppliers of dental equipment and supplies is included in Appendix C.

Golden Nuggets From the Experts

Nine diplomates of the American Veterinary Dental College offered their opinions on their own dental suites and advice for veterinarians getting started in the field of veterinary dentistry.

Jan Bellows at the All Pets Dental Clinic in Pembroke Pines, Florida

Dr. Bellows has three out of four treatment tables equipped for dentistry. He likes his intense light source and dislikes reaching for supplies. He would include suction as an important feature of the dental suite. When building a dental operatory, he recommends having the front of the treatment table fully accessible, with the anesthesia machine as part of the table, and having the treatment area well lighted.

Gregg DuPont at the Shoreline Veterinary Dental Clinic in Seattle

Dr. DuPont remodeled a separate room. He likes having his equipment and supplies within arm's reach, but finds his suite tends to be crowded. He recommends allowing for plenty of space between stations, with a remote compressor, good lighting, and a good music system. He suggests using the UC–Davis operatory as a template.

Edward Eisner of the Denver Veterinary Dental Service in Denver

Dr. Eisner moved his practice in 1993 and dedicated a portion of his treatment center as a dental operatory. He states that his favorite feature is the 5 feet of space he allowed between the two tables, making it comfortable to work. He likes his plaster trap and centralized wall-control panel for air and water. His biggest problem is poor tub drainage from the way the tables were installed. He suggests adding photography to your skills. It is a great marketing tool for promoting the benefits of dental care to your clients.

Steve Holmstrom of the Companion Animal Hospital in Belmont, California

Dr. Holmstrom's dental suite is in the treatment area of his busy hospital. He would prefer a separate room because of high noise levels. His equipment is within easy reach, and he uses a book of photos to index storage locations of dental supplies. He would like much more storage in his ideal suite, a shared X-ray station, and four tables. His golden nugget is "more storage and more counter space."

Thomas Kavanagh of the Village Animal Clinic in Farmington, Michigan

Dr. Kavanagh adapted a surgery suite for his dental operatory and likes his excellent lighting. His biggest problem is that his X-ray unit is not adaptable to his two tables, which is inconvenient. He would like overhead anesthesia delivery and overhead coil-less wiring to prevent tangles. He would remind the practitioner to refer cases to a specialist when the case is beyond his or her skill level.

Ken Lyon of the Mesa Veterinary Dental Service in Mesa, Arizona

Dr. Lyon uses a separate dental suite with two mobile tables. Having everything within arm's reach, including the computer system, is his favorite feature. He uses rolling carts and would prefer built-in storage and surface areas. He also would suggest using the UC-Davis dental suite, with its built-in features, as a template. Dr. Lyon's nugget is: "Think big! Design an area that you can grow into—one that has lots of cabinets and drawers and is comfortable and aesthetically pleasing, with good ventilation, and windows so you can see the real world every once in a while. Try to build in as much as you can to avoid cluttering up the area with anesthetic machines, tables, etc."

Tom Mulligan of the Main Street Small Animal Hospital in San Diego

Dr. Mulligan remodeled a double closet and has two dental operatories that are mirror images. He sits at the head of the table in an area about 36 inches deep and "is surrounded by all my toys." After four remodels, he is happy with his suite. Dr. Mulligan offers this sage advice, "Get ideas and do it right the first time!"

Frank Verstraete at the School of Veterinary Medicine of the University of California–Davis

Dr. Verstraete has the pleasure of using the much-admired Floyd Dental Suite. He likes the lighting, color scheme, Corian countertops, and sound system. He would like to have tables that adjust to height and tilt. One table is too close to the door and is difficult to use. He would add an X-ray reading area and computer workstation. He feels very fortunate to be able to work in this state-of-the-art facility.

Robert Wiggs of the Coit Road Animal Hospital in Dallas

Dr. Wiggs adapted a room for a single operatory and it now contains three. All of his anesthesia and dental delivery systems are built-in and he has excellent lighting. His biggest problem is the crowding he experiences in a room too small for his growing needs. He is currently making plans to expand his suite and improve his oral vacuum system. Dr. Wiggs states, "If you become really involved in dentistry, you will need more room than you think for all your toys."

Golden Nugget

Whether your dental suite is designed for entry-level dentistry or more advanced procedures, remember to allow for expansion both in quantity and quality. It is much easier to plan ahead for potential growth of the department than to add capacity later.

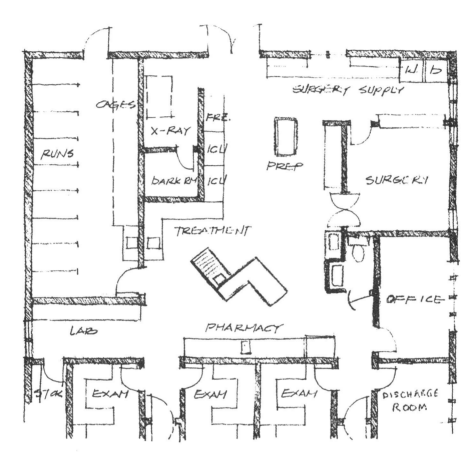

Figure 5-1   Sample Clinic Layout With Offset Treatment Tables.
Source: Veterinary Practice Building Design Starter Kit (Lakewood, Colo.: AAHA, 1990.)

The Physical Plant

A number of factors need to be considered when establishing the space where dental work will be performed.

Space Planning

For most practices, the dental department will be part of a multipurpose treatment room. The room is used for a wide range of nonsterile procedures, including contaminated surgeries, cleaning ears and teeth, and nail trims. It is the center of the activities of the hospital and can be hectic and noisy. Dental cases, especially the more advanced procedures, can be time consuming. More complex procedures require more equipment, supplies, and storage areas. Some sample treatment room floor plans are shown in Figures 5-1 through 5-7.

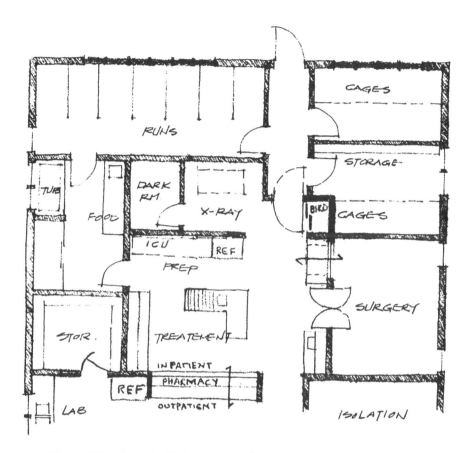

Figure 5-2 Sample Clinic Layout With L-Shaped Treatment Table.
Source: Veterinary Practice Building Design Starter Kit (Lakewood, Colo.: AAHA, 1990.)

Low Traffic

The dental suite should be located in a quiet alcove off the treatment area or in a separate room if possible (the ideal situation). The benefits of a separate room are reduced fomite levels and lower noise and activity levels to aid concentration. Having a separate room allows other procedures to progress without disturbing the dental team. Allow sufficient space for staff to move around the dental table. Through experience at our clinic, we have found that a minimum of 4 feet is necessary to work comfortably around a single table. Allow 5 feet if two tables are in use.

Adequate Counter and Storage Space

Dental procedures can require significant quantities of instruments and supplies. Plan to have two or three 4-square-foot counter surface areas within easy reach of the dental treatment table. A sink separate from the treatment table is important for washing instruments. While they are expensive, Corian countertops are easy to

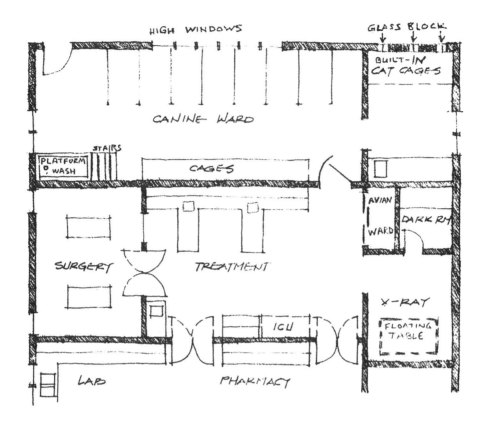

Figure 5-3   Sample Clinic Layout With Horseshoe Configuration.
Source: Veterinary Practice Building Design Starter Kit (Lakewood, Colo.: AAHA, 1990.)

maintain and resist staining. A horseshoe configuration offers the advantage of having a free end for the patient's head with adequate counter space for easy access to instruments and supplies. Rolling instrument carts make instruments available within arm's length. Countertops built at the standard standing height of 36 inches are more versatile than heights designed solely for dental use.

Lighting
Adequate lighting is required to illuminate the inside of the patient's mouth during dental procedures. Operating lights are available in incandescent, fluorescent, and halogen lamps, which provide different intensities and colors. A number of diplomates prefer a human dental light because it provides a softer light with less glare. Human dental lights can be purchased new or used from dental supply companies.

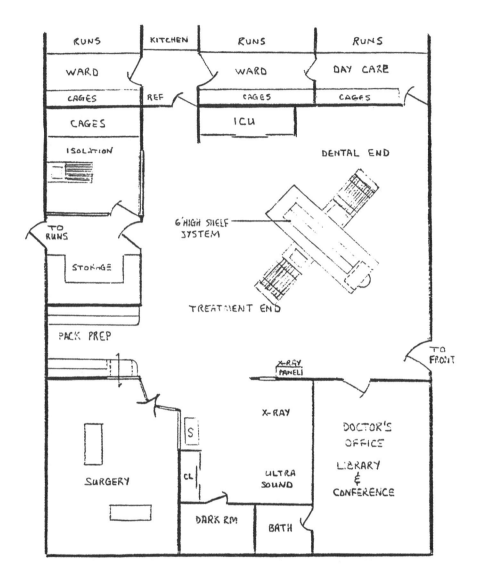

Figure 5-4   Sample Clinic Layout With Small Dental Area.
Source: Veterinary Practice Building Design Starter Kit (Lakewood, Colo.: AAHA, 1990.)

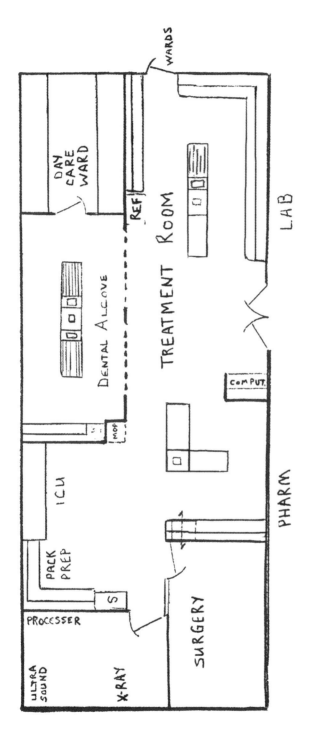

Figure 5-5   Sample Clinic Layout With Separate Dental Area.
Source: Veterinary Practice Building Design Starter Kit (Lakewood, Colo.: AAHA, 1990.)

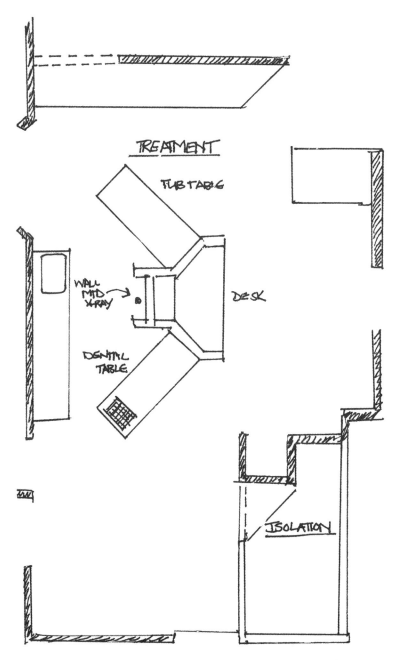

Figure 5-6   Sample Clinic Layout With Dental Table.
Courtesy of Front Range Veterinary Hospital, Ft. Collins, CO.

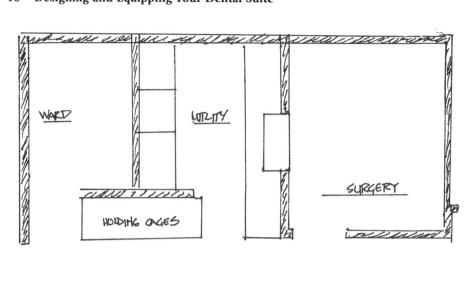

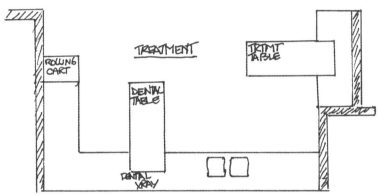

Figure 5-7   Sample Clinic Layout With Dental Area.
Courtesy of Campus Veterinary Clinic, Denver, CO.

Standard surgical procedure lights are also adequate for dental procedures.[2] There are also headlights and lights on fiberoptic handpieces for illuminating the dental field. What you choose is a matter of personal preference.

Electrical Outlets

Allow for electrical power needs when planning a dental operatory. Most dental and anesthesia monitoring equipment, as well as peripheral equipment such as circulating water pads and infusion pumps, requires an electrical outlet. It is efficient to have power strips installed to meet the electrical demands of dentistry. Generally, dental X-ray units sold in North America require 110 volts and should be wired to a dedicated circuit for consistent, high-quality results.

Dental Treatment Table with Water Supply and Drainage
Veterinarians are fortunate today because there are many options available when choosing a treatment table. Following are some features to consider when making your selection:

▲   **Water supply and drainage:** Using an ultrasonic or sonic scaler for dental prophylaxis requires a water source and method of removing excess water.

▲   **Knee space:** This is important for comfort when working. The dental scaler can be attached conveniently on the underside of the overhang and a rolling cart may be stored there when it is not in use.

▲   **Adjustability:** Some veterinarians prefer an adjustable-height table that can be placed at a slope for drainage.

▲   **Convenient storage and a number of drawers for dental supplies.**

One of the newest table designs, shown in Figure 5-8, is the Multi-Use Treatment Center from Shor-Line. The treatment center is a highly versatile work area designed with storage, countertop, and tub space. The buyer can combine up to three treatment tables with a shared utility center. The utility center contains plumbing, wiring, and oxygen lines and is a perfect location for procedure lights. The tables are available in eight configurations (see Figure 5-9) and can be added as your budget allows.[3] A "Roll-A-Bout" mobile storage unit is available that is a companion to Shor-Line's treatment tables (see Figure 5-10). The Suburban Surgical Company sells its Island Multi-Purpose Work Station with a wet and dry table. The wet table contains a rollout shelf to hold dental equipment and other supplies (see Figure 5-11). Also available, from X-ray Innovations, Inc. (Hollywood, Florida), is the Portable Prophy Table, constructed of heavy-duty plastic with water collection tray as an inexpensive alternative. The unit has a slight incline for proper positioning and removable drain and sink for easy cleanup.

Auxiliary Equipment
The following are used in conjunction with the treatment table.

▲   **Adjustable-height stool with back support.**

▲   **Rolling storage carts:** These provide additional counter space and storage. Carts are available from Shor-Line® (Kansas City, Missouri) in plastic laminate; less expensive plastic carts can be purchased from catalogs such as Medical Arts Press (Minneapolis, Minneapolis) and discount department stores.

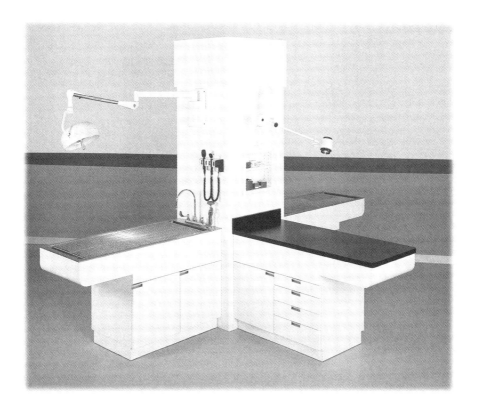

Figure 5-8   Multi-Use Treatment Center.
From Shor-Line Catalog, 1998, Kansas City, MO.

Anesthesia Delivery System and Monitoring Capability

Gas anesthetic maintenance is ideal for dentistry because the patients should be already intubated to prevent aspiration of water and calculus debris. Either isoflurane or sevoflurane gas is ideal for dental procedures. Gas anesthesia offers rapid induction and recovery for veterinary patients. One of your client's primary concerns is the risk of complications from anesthesia, and offering the safest gas available is performing the best service for your patients and their owners. Wall-mounted, over-the-patient units are convenient because they extend out from the wall for use and reduce the clutter in the work area. Monitoring the patient with respiratory monitors, pulse oximeters, and blood pressure or EKG monitors is important for patient safety. For staff safety, the AAHA recommends an active gas scavenging system to remove exhaust anesthetic gases.

FOR EACH LOCATION 1, 2, & 3 CHOOSE TUB OR TABLE WITH CABINET TYPE FROM
CHART BELOW (A-H) OR CHOOSE NONE. THEN CHOOSE EXTRA OPTIONS FOR EACH
LOCATION FROM EXTRA OPTION CHART (J-L).

CHOOSE FOR EACH LOCATION												
LOCATION	NONE	A	B	C	D	E	F	G	H	J	K	L
1												
2												
3												

EXTRA OPTIONS:
J	NONE
K	PULL-OUT SHELF W/GLIDE BRACKETS
L	DOORS ON BOTH SIDES OF CABINET

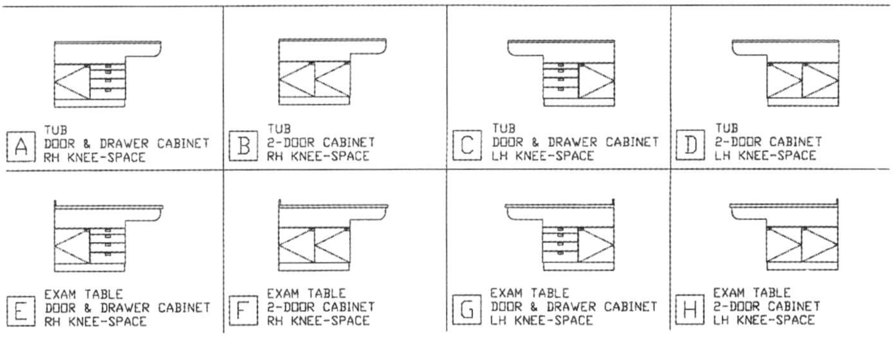

A — TUB DOOR & DRAWER CABINET RH KNEE-SPACE
B — TUB 2-DOOR CABINET RH KNEE-SPACE
C — TUB DOOR & DRAWER CABINET LH KNEE-SPACE
D — TUB 2-DOOR CABINET LH KNEE-SPACE
E — EXAM TABLE DOOR & DRAWER CABINET RH KNEE-SPACE
F — EXAM TABLE 2-DOOR CABINET RH KNEE-SPACE
G — EXAM TABLE DOOR & DRAWER CABINET LH KNEE-SPACE
H — EXAM TABLE 2-DOOR CABINET LH KNEE-SPACE

FOR EACH SIDE A, B, C, & D CHOOSE OPTION FROM
CHART BELOW (1-5). THEN CHOOSE EXTRA OPTIONS
FROM EXTRA OPTION CHART (6-8).

CHOOSE FOR EACH SIDE								
SIDE	1	2	3	4	5	6	7	8
A								
B								
C								
D								

EXTRA OPTIONS:
6	NONE
7	DOOR WITHOUT LOCK
8	DOOR WITH LOCK

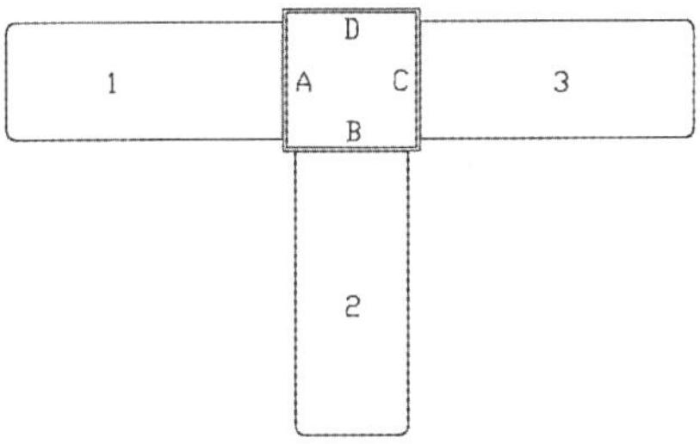

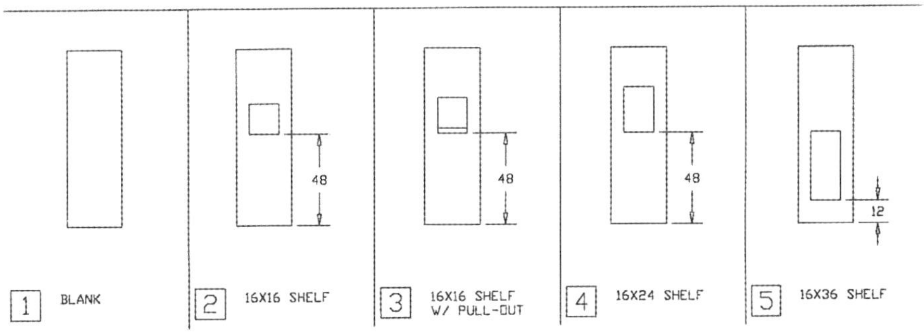

1 BLANK
2 16X16 SHELF — 48
3 16X16 SHELF W/ PULL-OUT — 48
4 16X24 SHELF — 48
5 16X36 SHELF — 12

Figure 5-9 Dental Treatment Center Configurations.
From Shor-Line Catalog, 1998, Kansas City, MO.

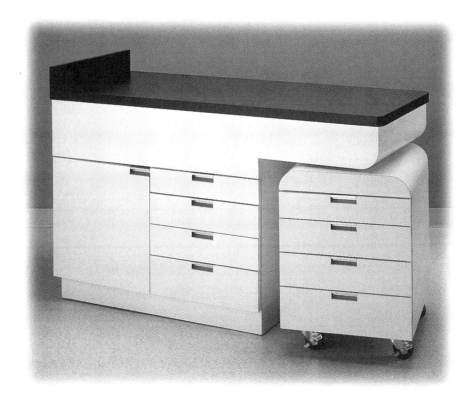

Figure 5-10   Mobile Dental Cart With Exam Table.
From Shor-Line Catalog, 1998, Kansas City, MO.

Dental Radiography

The ability to expose dental radiographs is essential for proper diagnosis and treatment of dental problems. Whether a tooth can be salvaged or should be extracted is often determined by dental radiography. Intra-oral dental films can be taken with the standard veterinary medical unit by collimating down to the size of dental film, but this procedure requires moving the patient to the machine, which may be inconvenient if it has to be done on a regular basis. An intra-oral x-ray unit that extends from the wall or ceiling will make positioning and exposing dental films much easier. The newer machines feature reduced scatter with clearer images, and dental film is inexpensive. Used dental X-ray units are also available but should be purchased with caution. If you are considering a used unit, be certain to purchase it from a reputable dealer who knows where the unit came from and why it was replaced.

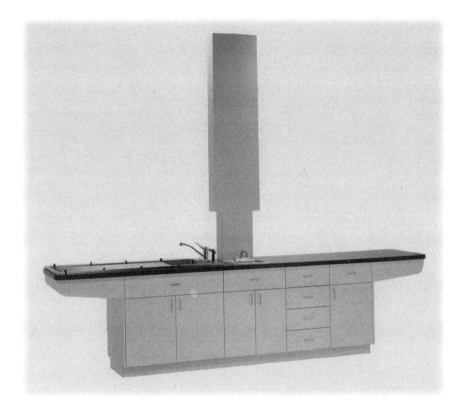

Figure 5-11 Multi-Purpose Workstation.
Courtesy of Suburban Surgical Company, Inc., Wheeling, IL.

Dental Equipment and Supplies

To provide dental services, certain equipment is basic and essential. Choosing the equipment that meets budgetary and performance criteria can be challenging. This section presents a brief discussion of the dental equipment required for dental prophylaxis and advanced dental procedures. The authors of several recent books have discussed equipment and supplies in great depth, and I advise you to consult those books for more detailed information.[4] Supplies and equipment necessary for routine dental prophylaxis can be purchased from most veterinary suppliers. The estimated prices listed in the following sections were those that were in effect in October 1998. When preparing to perform advanced dental procedures, it may be necessary to use a human dental supplier. Human dentists may be your best resource for information about local suppliers and repair service. A list of dental equipment manufacturers and suppliers appears in Appendix C.

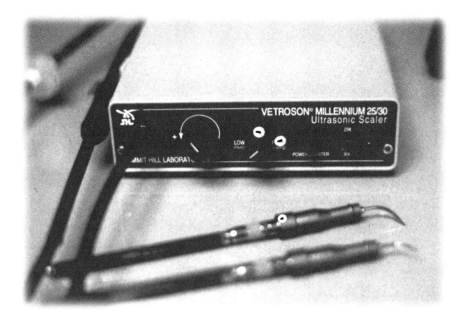

Figure 5-12   Ultrasonic Dental Scaler.
Courtesy of Summit Hill Laboratories, Navesink, NJ.

Dental Prophylaxis

The purpose of this section is to help you equip your hospital with the tools necessary to perform high-quality dental prophylaxis. Approximate prices are included for this equipment; these often fall into broad ranges. Generally, the lower priced machines will tend to be less powerful, less versatile, and less dependable than the more expensive units. Depending on your volume, it is a good idea to purchase the highest quality piece of equipment in your price range. A better quality machine will pay for itself many times over with increased production and minimal downtime. For a detailed, step-by-step description of performing dental prophylaxis, please refer to dental textbooks, such as *Veterinary Dental Techniques* by Holmstrom, Frost, and Eisner (Philadelphia: W.B. Saunders, 1998).

Ultrasonic and Sonic Scalers

The ultrasonic dental scaler (Figure 5-12) is the backbone of veterinary dentistry. A scaler is used to remove the plaque and tartar from teeth by vibrating off the accumulated material with sound waves. Both ultrasonic and sonic scalers work in a similar manner using "mechanical kick" to remove calculus and the water spray to cavitate or clean the tooth surface.[5] Two key issues in the use of scalers are staff

training and maintenance. The scalers will operate better and require less maintenance when the staff is properly trained in the use of the machine. Following are
descriptions of various scalers.

1. **Ultrasonic scalers** vibrate at a speed of 19,000–45,000 cycles per second.
   Generally, the higher speed units provide a shorter working time. They are
   electrically operated and most models require the use of a water supply because
   they generate heat and must use a water spray to cool the teeth. There is the risk
   of heat damage to the tooth and surrounding tissues if the machine is used
   incorrectly. Dental scalers are durable and require little maintenance. There are
   three types of ultrasonic scalers (see Table 5-1).[6] The magnetostrictive and
   ferromagnetostrictive machines use metal stacks and tips that will wear out and
   break. The piezoelectric scaler employs a silver-coated crystal that vibrates the
   tip in a curved linear pattern. The tips are half as expensive as other types of
   scalers, but tend to require replacement twice as often.

2. **Sonic scalers** operate with pressurized air passing through the shaft of the
   handpiece, causing it to oscillate in an oval-elliptical pattern. They operate at a
   slower speed of 8,000–18,000 cps and require a compressor for pressurized air,
   nitrogen, or CO_2 source. If you plan to use a sonic scaler, a 1 hp or bigger compressor will be needed to handle the workload. These scalers are popular in
   human dentistry because they are slower and quieter, use less water, and vibrate
   less against the teeth. Because veterinary patients are normally anesthetized
   during the procedure, these considerations are less important than in human
   dentistry.

3. **Rotary scalers** are high-speed, six-sided burs that fit on a handpiece of an air-
   driven dental unit. These burs operate at speeds in excess of 100,000 rpm and
   can be used to vibrate calculus loose. They should be used with extreme caution
   because of the potential for damage to the tooth and surrounding tissues.

Table 5-1   Types of Ultrasonic Scalers

Type of Scaler	Action	Frequency (cycles per sec)	Price Range/Advantages
Magnetostrictive (i.e., Cavitron or similar, Vetroson)	Figure eight	25,000–30,000	$600–1,000 2 speed, economical, auto-tuning, accessory irrigator
Piezoelectric (i.e., Star-tec, Spartan)	Linear	40,000	$750 faster, less damage to tooth surface
Ferromagnetostrictive (i.e., Odontoson)	Circular	42,000	$1,300–1,800 faster, can use irrigating solutions, can be used for periodontal treatment with additional tips

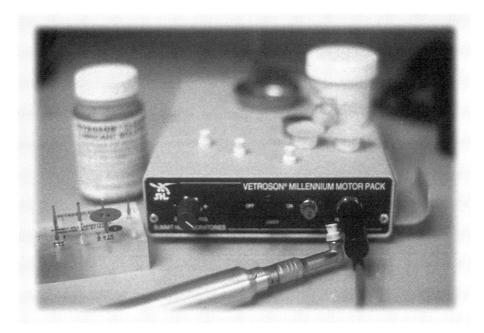

Figure 5-13   Dental Polisher.
Courtesy of Summit Hill Laboratories, Navesink, NJ.

Dental Polishers

The vibrating action of the scaler causes microetching on the surface of the tooth. If the teeth are not polished after cleaning, the surface will be slightly roughened and will promote the rapid formation of plaque and calculus. The process of polishing delays the onset by smoothing the microetches, thus increasing the interval between dental care visits. Polishing the teeth adds value to your dental services, because your clients will appreciate your efforts to lengthen the time period between professional cleanings. Polishing can be performed with a small electrical engine (Figure 5-13) designed for this use, costing approximately $200–800. If you have a dental delivery system or plan to purchase one, a prophy angle can be attached to an air-powered slow-speed handpiece at an expense of $15–250. Prophy paste should be used as a lubricant to avoid heating the tooth. A Dentalaire mobile dental delivery system with separate sonic scaler is shown in Figure 5-14; it costs approximately $1,600–3,000.

Hand Instruments

In addition to the scaler, you will need a selection of hand instruments for tooth extraction, gross calculus removal, and hand scaling of the supra- and subgingival tooth surfaces. There is a large variety of instruments and much of your selection will depend on personal preference. It is important to inspect the instrument for damage

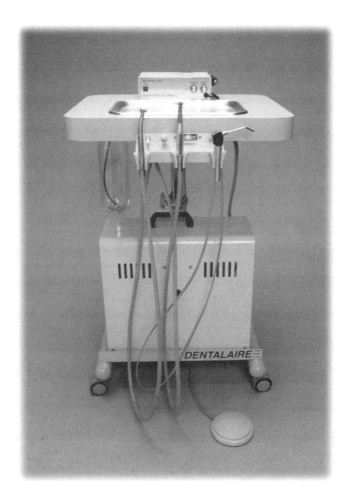

Figure 5-14   Mobile Dental Cart With Scaler.
Courtesy of Dentalaire, Fountain Valley, CA.

after each use to prevent injuring the patient. The number of instruments you should have in your inventory depends on your volume. The curettes and scalers will require sharpening about every third use. It is convenient to have enough instruments to reduce sharpening maintenance to once a week. Shown in Table 5-2 is a brief list of the more commonly used hand instruments.

Dental X-Ray Unit

Veterinary dental specialists believe that a dental X-ray unit is required equipment because the proper treatment for a tooth sometimes cannot be determined without a diagnostic X-ray. The advantages of a dental radiography unit over a

Table 5-2   Commonly Used Hand Instruments

Instrument	Purpose	Price
Calculus removal forceps (large and small size)	Efficiently remove large deposits of calculus	$36
Dental hoe or chisel	Strong instrument for gross calculus removal	$10–20
Dental claw	Remove gross calculus	$10–20
Fine hand scalers: Jacquette 2Y-3Y, Universal, etc.	Remove deposits above the gumline	$8–25
Curettes: Gracey, etc.	Remove calculus and fibrotic deposits above and below the gumline	$20
Periodontal probes	Measure the gingival pocket depth	$17
Periodontal explorers	Detect surface irregularities	$5–10
Dental mirrors	Visualize difficult-to-see areas	$16
Surgical elevators	In extractions, break the periodontal ligament and displace the root from the alveolar socket	$10–85
Periosteal elevator	Used in gingival flap surgery	$20
Extraction forceps	Grasp the tooth, remove gross calculus	$25
Root tip pick	Retrieve fractured root tips	$8

standard veterinary medical machine are convenience, economics, and high-quality images. A machine located at the dental treatment table is quick and easy to use and the film is economical to purchase. These low-milliamperage units use parallel x-rays and a smaller focal spot, yielding higher quality diagnostic films. The machines can be purchased new or used, but caution should be exercised when considering the purchase of a used machine. The price can range from $1,500 for a good, used unit to $5,500 for a new standard unit. Most of the newer machines are compatible with digital X-ray format. Dental machines come with a standard 72-inch arm, and it is also possible to order an 84-inch arm. Seventy-two inches is the minimum length required for all dentistry and the longer arm is necessary if you plan to access the unit from two treatment tables. The Image Vet 70 (AFP Imaging Corporation, Elmsford, N.Y.) is a mobile dental X-ray unit designed specifically for small animal dentistry; the control dial has settings for canines and felines.

Dental film is small and economical to purchase. Each individual film is protected by a light-proof cover and does not require a cassette or darkroom to use. Consult Appendix C for a list of suppliers.

Dental films may be processed manually or with an automatic processor. The easiest and most economical method is to use a *chairside darkroom*, which is a self-contained, lightproof, countertop unit that contains four small cups for chemicals and rinse water. It features a see-through lid and diaphragm hand and wrist apertures that make it possible for the operator to observe while developing the film. The

Table 5-3   Expendable Supplies Used in a Sample Dental Prophylaxis

Supplies Used	Cost
Endotracheal tube ($4.37 per tube; 5 uses per tube)	$ .87 per use
Anesthetic medications (isoflurane @ $10/hr, ketamine, diazepam, glyccopyrralate)	13.00 per patient
Syringes and needles	.50 each
Scaler x 2	1.00 per use
Curette x 2	1.00 per use
Towels – to cushion head and protect eyes	.10 per use
Periodontal probe	.50 per use
Polishing cup	.20 each
Prophy paste – 2 cups	.15
Gauze sponges – 20 3" x 3" sponges	.20
Mouth rinse (CET Chx solution, Viadent, etc.)	.50
Curved tip syringe for flushing	.40
Exam gloves, mask	.30
Paper towel or gauze to collect debris and water	.10
Total cost	**$18.82**

chemicals are two-step rapid processing solutions. When rinsed, films are hung from small hangers to dry and are then stored in cardboard or plastic film mounts. The chairside darkroom costs approximately $250 and the chemicals are $25 for a pair of developer and fixer quarts. Dental films may also be developed with an automatic processor, but there are disadvantages of cost, time, and risk of losing films.

Expendable Supplies

With any procedure, expendable supplies will be used in the process. The supplies used in a typical hour-long dental prophylaxis for a 60-pound dog are listed in Table 5-3. The amounts of drugs and supplies will vary according to size, species, and extent of cleaning required.

Advanced Dental Procedures

The next step beyond providing basic dental prophylaxis is to add periodontal treatment and basic endodontic therapy. Many of your patients will present with a fractured tooth that can be salvaged with a root canal treatment. The patient will benefit by being relieved of oral pain and the risk of future abscesses and by having the continued use of the treated tooth. The practice will benefit from the increased good will of the client and the income from providing advanced dental services. To offer these services, some additional equipment is required. The selection of equipment will depend on considerations such as budget, the volume and character of the dental caseload, and space available for equipment.

Dental Delivery System

A dental delivery unit is a highly versatile piece of equipment that can be used to polish teeth when finishing prophylaxis and for many aspects of advanced dentistry. The least expensive units have electrically driven motors. They are small and portable and require less maintenance, but they are also less efficient and prone to mechanical breakdown. The fastest and most effective systems are air-driven units powered by a source of pressurized gas with a regulator, control box, and handpieces. The source of gas can be a tank of pressurized carbon dioxide or nitrogen or an air compressor. The power is delivered to the handpieces by means of tubing connected to the air source. The air, along with water, is used to cool the handpiece, cutting bur, and tooth during the procedure. Air-driven units can be mounted on a mobile cart or stand (see Figure 5-14), on a wall-mounted extension arm, as an over-the-patient unit, or as a small countertop unit. The price can range from $500 to more than $10,000, depending on the features required. A wall-mounted system costs $3,000 to $4,000. The purchase of a dental delivery system is a complex decision that depends on the present needs and future goals of the practice. A complete discussion of the advantages and disadvantages of various types of systems can be found in other references.[7] It is my intention only to expose you to the possibilities. Following are some features to consider when purchasing a dental delivery system.

1. **Compressor:** The compressor is a source of pressurized gas to operate the handpieces. Its strength is measured in horsepower. Compressors can be either tableside, on the same stand or cart as the console, or in a remote location. Most compressors contain oil as a coolant and require monitoring and maintenance. The tableside compressors are usually less powerful ($1/2$ hp) and can be used only at one station at a time. They are useful for procedures of less than approximately 30 minutes in duration. The noise level of the compressor is a major factor to consider when selecting a tableside unit. Whisper-quiet compressors are available. Remote compressors can be located apart from the dental operatory, which will reduce the noise and clutter. The remote units are generally 1 hp or larger and can be used to power multiple workstations. A cautionary note: The power or speed of a handpiece is reduced as the distance from the compressor is increased.[8]

2. **Handpieces and control panel:** Handpieces are the instruments that are used to perform advanced dental procedures. The control panel is necessary to adjust air and water pressure for each handpiece.

    ▲   **Low-speed handpiece:** This handpiece is used for polishing with a prophy angle and for specialized instruments requiring slower speeds and higher torques. It usually operates at 4,000–25,000 rpm and can be used to section a multirooted tooth for extraction and to finish restorations.

▲   **High-speed handpiece:** This is used for rapid cutting of teeth and bone. The high-speed handpiece operates at speeds up to 400,000 rpm. (Caveat: The speed at the compressor may be 400,000 rpm, but it is often approximately 100,000 rpm when it reaches the handpiece.) The high-speed handpiece is used for dental access and cavity and crown preparation. Water cooling protects the handpiece and tooth from the heat generated. The low torque allows stalling, which prevents teeth from shattering. Fiberoptic handpieces are available that illuminate the operating site.

3. **Sonic scaler:** This is an optional device that allows the technician to perform dental prophylaxis. It is a handpiece powered by an air delivery system.

4. **Three-way air/water syringe:** The three-way syringe is used to irrigate the gingival sulcus, rinse the oral cavity, cool the tooth, and dry it before installing surface restorations.

5. **Variable speed foot control:** This device allows the operator to work without having to use a manual switch, thus freeing the hands.

Electrosurgery Unit

Oral tissues are well supplied with blood and tend to heal quickly. An electrosurgery unit is useful for controlling hemorrhage during periodontal surgery and tumor removal. Having a unit available can promote efficiency and reduce procedure time.

Irrigation and Suction

It is helpful to have a method of irrigating the tissues and flushing away debris and blood during dental procedures. The three-way air/water syringe should be purchased with your dental delivery system. Suction capability is also available as an option on some delivery systems or as a separate unit.

Hand Instruments and Expendable Supplies

A large variety of instrumentation and supplies can be used in advanced dental procedures. It is beyond the scope of this guidebook to attempt to list all of the possible items needed for each procedure, but recent textbooks do offer extensive information on the subject.[9] It is also possible to purchase kits that are useful for initial procedures from some supply houses (for example, Dr. Shipp's Laboratories, Beverly Hills, Calif., and Cislak Manufacturing, Glenview, Ill., offer periodontal kits; see Appendix C for addresses). After using a kit, you can decide which instruments work best in your hands and adjust your inventory accordingly. The speakers at dental seminars routinely offer lists of instruments and supplies that are useful for the procedures they discuss.

Ergonomics

Ergonomics is defined as the study of the efficiency of persons in their work environment.[10] To expand upon this, efficiency is affected when staff members develop physical ailments as a result of performing their duties. When designing a dental operatory, attention should be devoted to the health and safety of the staff members who will be performing the services. As the numbers of your dental procedures increase, so will the risk of repetitive stress injuries to staff members. There are a number of other cumulative trauma disorders (CTD), the most common being carpal tunnel syndrome. Improper posture, incorrect handling of dental instruments, and poorly designed dental treatment areas cause most of these injuries.

The incidence of CTD injuries can be reduced by a number of preventive actions. Following are some considerations to keep in mind when designing your dental operatory:

▲ **Chair or stool:** The chair should be of adjustable height so that the operator can avoid hunching over the patient and bending or twisting the neck. The chair should have an adjustable backrest and five castors for stability and mobility. If the employee's feet cannot touch the floor, a sloping footrest should be provided.

▲ **Kneehole:** The treatment table should be cantilevered to allow at least 16 vertical inches for legroom. There should be 24 inches in front of the feet for movement and stretching.

▲ **Work area:** The patient should be positioned so that the operator's elbow is horizontally even with the patient's mouth. Adjustable height or tilting tables can be useful for reducing fatigue. The instruments, supplies, and controls for the equipment should be within easy reach.

▲ **Operator's posture and movement:** The staff and clinician should be trained in the proper use of the equipment and instruments. Holding and using a hand instrument incorrectly can lead to muscle fatigue. In a seated position, the operator should maintain a 90° angle at the knees and hip joints, using foot and back rests if necessary. The hands and elbows should be lower than the shoulders to maintain relaxed shoulders and neck. The operator should vary the movements of the hands and fingers to avoid strain. Physical therapists also recommend taking regular breaks to stretch for 10–15 seconds to increase circulation and allow for muscle recovery.[11] These actions may be helpful to prevent repetitive stress injuries.

▲ **High-quality equipment:** Better equipment will generally be designed for easier use. With proper maintenance of the equipment and instruments, they will function at optimal levels and allow the dental team to complete the procedures more quickly and efficiently. Sharp instruments reduce fatigue and procedure time.

Worker Safety

The use of high-speed dental equipment and ultrasonic scalers causes aerosols of bacteria and debris to be sprayed into the dental operatory environment. Without protection, the staff is exposed to potentially infectious bacteria that can cause upper respiratory disease that can be communicable to other staff members and clients. Flying debris may cause injury to unprotected eyes and result in eye infection. Chemicals, sharp instruments, and lights pose other risks as well. The use of personal protective equipment should be required for all staff members who work in the dental operatory. All staff members operating ultrasonic scalers and other high-speed equipment should wear eye protection, surgical mask, latex gloves, and hair coverings. Disposable masks are available with a protective eye shield attached to the mask from suppliers that specialize in dental equipment (for example, Safti-shield, Henry Schein, Inc., Melville, N.Y.). When exposing dental X-ray films, the staff should leave the area or wear protective lead clothing.[12]

The topic of worker safety has been explored very briefly in this chapter. In addition to personal protective equipment, other safety issues that go beyond the dental department should be addressed in all veterinary hospitals. A program should be in place for compliance with the standards and regulations of the Occupational Safety and Health Administration.

References

1. M. R. Hafen, "State-of-the-Art Design: Put It to Work for You," in *Supplement to Veterinary Economics* (February 1993): 18.
2. D. Ludwig, "Keeping Pace with Changes in Dental Suite Design," *Veterinary Economics* (February 1996): 80.
3. Shor-Line Catalog 1998, Kansas City, Mo., 1998: D7.
4. S. E. Holmstrom, P. Frost, and E. R. Eisner, *Veterinary Dental Techniques* 2d ed. (Philadelphia: W.B. Saunders, 1998): 31–106; R. B. Wiggs and H. B. Lobprise, *Veterinary Dentistry—Principles & Practice* (Philadelphia: Lippincott-Raven, 1997): 1–54; C. Harvey and P. P. Emily, *Small Animal Dentistry* (St. Louis, Mo.: Mosby-Year Book, 1993): 378–400.
5. Wiggs and Lobprise, *Veterinary Dentistry—Principles & Practice,* 16–17.
6. Holmstrom, Frost, and Eisner, *Veterinary Dental Techniques,* 2d ed.: 58–59.
7. Holstrom, Frost, and Eisner, *Veterinary Dental Techniques,* 2d ed.: ch. 2; Wiggs and Lobprise, *Veterinary Dentistry—Principles & Practice*: chs. 1 and 2; Harvey and Emily, *Small Animal Dentistry*: ch. 11.
8. Holstrom, Frost, and Eisner, *Veterinary Dental Techniques,* 2d ed.: 34–35.
9. Holstrom, Frost, and Eisner, *Veterinary Dental Techniques,* 2d ed.: ch. 2; Wiggs and Lobprise, *Veterinary Dentistry—Principles & Practice*: chs. 1 and 2; Harvey and Emily, *Small Animal Dentistry*: ch. 11.
10. *Oxford Dictionary and Thesaurus, American Edition* (New York: The Oxford University Press, 1996): 489.
11. C. Kauder, "Ergonomically Correct," *Rocky Mountain News* [Denver, Colo.], March 23, 1999: 3D–4D.
12. Holstrom, Frost, and Eisner, *Veterinary Dental Techniques,* 2d ed.: 505.

CHAPTER 6

The Paperwork: Keeping Dental Records and Setting Your Fees

Designing Your Dental Records

Dental formulas vary substantially among the different species of animals in both large and small animal medicine. It is important to record in detail the results of the dental examination and the treatment performed on each tooth. Developing specialized dental forms for each species that you treat will facilitate the handling of your dental cases. Photographic documentation and digital imaging can enhance your dental recordkeeping. Furthermore, having complete documentation of each case with your client's informed consent will help protect you and your practice legally.

When designing your dental records, you may wish to use the Problem Oriented Medical Record system and list "SOAP" (subjective, objective, assessment, and plan) information to describe each problem. This is a logical and convenient format that clearly describes the entering complaint and your treatment strategy. The record should be easy for a person less knowledgeable in the field to read and understand. Whether you choose this format or another, a dental record should include the following items:

1. **Clinic, client, and patient information.**
2. **Date of the visit.**
3. **Chief complaint:** This section should consist of subjective, historical information as described by the client about the patient, including diet, home oral hygiene, and other relevant information. Listing the client's reason for the visit ensures that the entering complaint is addressed in the treatment plan.
4. **General medical and dental observation:** This includes objective information such as the results of laboratory testing and the physical and oral examinations.
5. **Dental anatomical charts with a tooth identification system and key to abbreviations used:** Dental diagrams allow you to quickly note in detail the pre- and posttreatment status of each tooth.

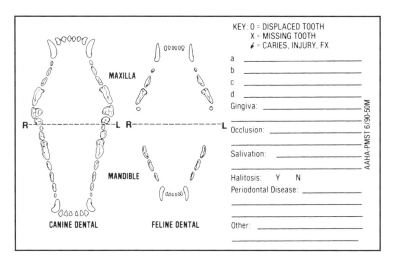

Figure 6-1   AAHA Self-Adhesive Dental Chart.

6. **Assessment or diagnosis:** In addition to your assessment, this section may include photographs, radiographs, digital imaging, and consultations with specialists.

7. **Plan and treatment:** The treatment protocol should be described on the dental record along with the prognosis and recommendations to the client. Anesthetics and other medications should also be noted in this section.

Dental forms may come in the form of self-adhesive labels purchased from the AAHA (see Figure 6-1) or from other sources. Rubber or self-inking stamps may also be used for basic recordkeeping. Using whole-page forms designed specifically for dentistry will streamline your operations and allow you to record the case in greater detail. The format may be fill-in-the-blank or a checklist. Samples of the fill-in-the-blank for canines and felines are shown in Figures 6-2 through 6-5. An example of the checklist format is shown in Figure 6-6. In addition to these examples, *Instructions for Veterinary Clients,* by David Erlewein and Eugene Kuhns, includes dental charts for dogs and cats.[1] Veterinary software programs such as IDEXX Informatics Better Choice and Cornerstone products have incorporated this book into their systems, and instructions may be individualized for your clients.

In addition to maintaining dental records on paper, you may also store dental information in your computer. Digital imaging technology can allow you to photograph the oral cavity and scan the results into your computer for e-mailing or client communications. Pre- and posttreatment photographs offer a visual record of the presenting condition and results of the treatment. Digital imaging is a new and rapidly expanding technology that is becoming more commonly used in general practice.

Page ______

EDWARD R. EISNER, D.V.M.
Diplomate, Amer. Vet. Dental College
Campus Veterinary Clinic, P.C.
2186 South Colorado Boulevard, Suite C
Denver, Colorado 80222
Phone (303) 757-8481 FAX (303) 759-4729

DENVER VETERINARY DENTAL SERVICE

CANINE

Date: ______________

Owner & NO. ______________
Name ______________ Breed ______________
Birth Date __________ Sex ______ Color _____
Referred by: ______________

Reason for Visit ______________ Diet: ______________
Previous Dental History ______________
Home Dental Care: Brushing ______________ Oral Rinse ____________ Medication ______________
Other Pertinent History ______________
NPO ________ HRS.

EXAMINATION (Gen. Cond. _________ ; Weight ________lbs; Heart __________ Color________ CRT_______)
☐ No Teeth Missing

TREATMENT: VT _____ DVM _________

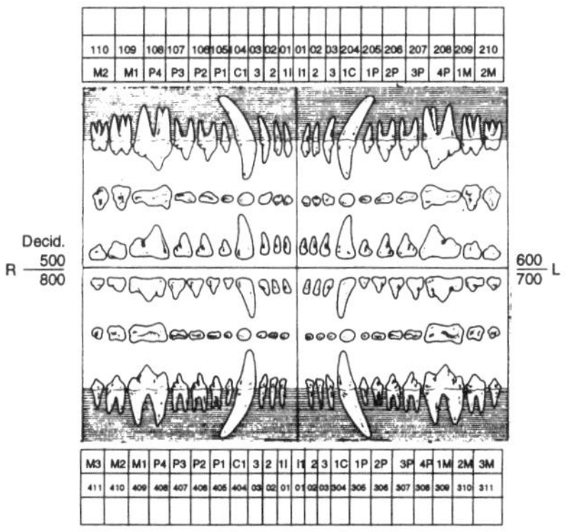

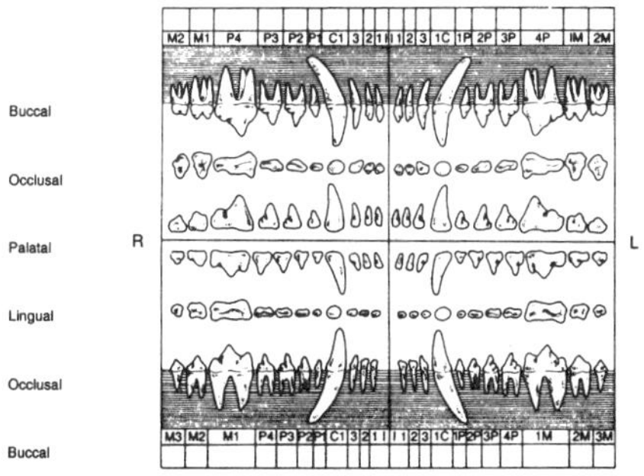

KEY: 0 = Normal 1 = Mild 2 = Moderate 3 = Advanced

AL	Attachment Loss	FEN/FIS	Fenestration / Fistula	O	Missing Tooth	RL/IR/RR	Resorptive Lesion/ Int. Resorpion/ Root Resorption
CA	Caries	Fx O/C	Fractured Tooth Open / Closed	OM	Oral Mass		
CI	Calculus Index (0-3)			ONF	Oronasal Fistula		
CU	Contact Ulcer	GH	Gingival Hyperplasia	OST	Osteomyelitis	S/I/E	Staining Intrinsic/Extrinsic
CR	Crowded Tooth	GI	Gingival Index (0-3)	P(mm)	Perio.Pkt. (mm)	STM	Stomatitis
DC	Dentigerous Cyst	GR	Gingival Recession	PA	Periapical Bone Lysis	SUP	Supernumerary
E	Enamel Defect	IR	Internal Resorption	ROT	Rotated Tooth	SYM/S	Symphysis Separation
EP	Epulis	LFD	Lip Fold Dermatitis	RD/R	Retained Deciduous Tooth / Root	TA/TL	Tooth Avulsion/Luxation
F	Furcation 1(v), 2(>), 3(>)	-->	Malpositioned tooth direction			VT/NV	Vital Tooth/Nonvital
FB	Foreign Body	M	Mobile Tooth (1-3)			W	Worn Tooth

TREATMENT KEY

BE/I	Biopsy Excisional / Incisional	IL/OL	Inlay / OnLay	P&FS	Pit & Fissure Sealer	RX	Root Extraction
BFR	Buccal Fold Removal	IO	Interceptive Orthodontics	PS	Perio Surgery	VP	Vital Pulpotomy
BR	Bridge	OA/I/A/R	Orthodontic Appliance Install / Adjust / Removal	PSP	Perio Splint	WW	Wait & Watch
CM/PFM	Crown Metal/ Porcelain Fused to Metal			RA/C/I	Restoration Amalgam / Composite / Ionomer	X/XS/XSS	Extraction / Hemisect / Sx.Ext
		OE	Occlusal Equilibration				
FAR/GG/LS/RB	Apical/ FGing.Graft / Lat.Slid / Rev.Bev.	OI/W	Osseous Implant / Wiring	RC	Root Canal Tmt.		
		OP	Odontoplasty	RCS	Root Canal Surgical		
FG / FV	Fluoride Gell / Varnish	PC	Pulp Cap	RPC/O	Root Planing Closed / Open		

Occlusal Evaluation:

Oral Examination (Saliva, Breath, Tonsils, Lnn):

Periodontal Evaluation:

Gingival Index: (GI) 0 = Normal, No Swelling. 1 = No Bleeding When Probed 2 = Bleeds When Probed 3 = Spontaneous Bleeding

Calculus Index: (CI) 0 = No Plaque 1 = Soft Film at Margin 2 = Calculus Easily Seen 3 = Heavy Deposits

Endodontic Evaluation:

Radiographic Evaluation:

TREATMENT PLAN:

LIAISON WITH REFERRING DOCTOR

Person contacted	Phone	Record	Person

ANESTHESIA	TIME	DOSE	AGENT
Preanesthetic			
Anesth. Induct.			

E. T. size __________GAS________
End of Procedure ________
Support ______________

PROPHYLAXIS Home Care Instructions ______________

1. Ultrasonic cleaning ____________
2. Subgingival curettage ____________
3. Polishing ____________
4. Other ______________

ASSESSMENT/ADDITIONAL THERAPY:

Figure 6-2 Canine Fill-in-the-Blank Dental Chart.
Courtesy of Campus Veterinary Clinic, P.C., Denver, CO.

Page ______

EDWARD R. EISNER, D.V.M.
Diplomate, Amer. Vet. Dental College
Campus Veterinary Clinic, P.C.
2186 South Colorado Boulevard, Suite C
Denver, Colorado 80222
Phone (303) 757-8481 FAX (303) 759-4729

DENVER VETERINARY DENTAL SERVICE
FELINE

Date: ________________

Owner & NO. ______________________
Name ______________ Breed ___________
Birth Date _________ Sex ______ Color _____
Referred by: ______________________

Reason for Visit ______________________________________ Diet: ______________
Previous Dental History ______________________________________
Home Dental Care: Brushing ____________________ Oral Rinse ___________ Medication ____________
Other Pertinent History ______________________________________
NPO ________ HRS.

EXAMINATION (Gen. Cond. _________ ; Weight _________lbs; Heart __________ Color_______ CRT_______)
☐ No Teeth Missing

TREATMENT: VT _____ DVM _________

Decid.
R 500/800

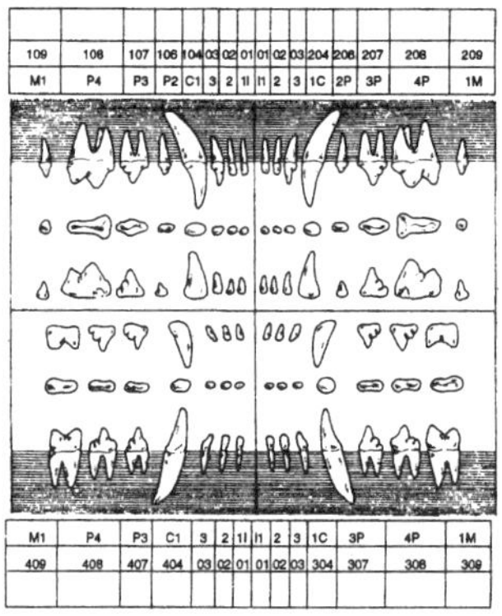

600/700 L

Buccal
Occlusal
Palatal
Lingual
Occlusal
Buccal

R

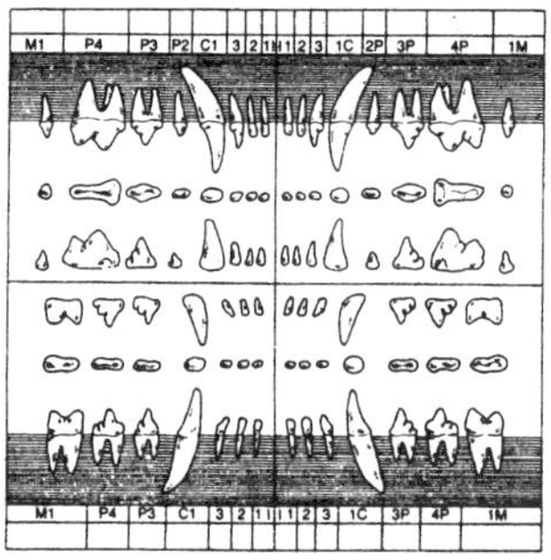

L

KEY: 0 = Normal 1 = Mild 2 = Moderate 3 = Advanced

AL	Attachment Loss	FEN/FIS	Fenestration / Fistula	O	Missing Tooth	RL/IR/RR	Resorptive Lesion/ Int. Resorpion/ Root Resorption
CA	Caries	Fx O/C	Fractured Tooth Open / Closed	OM	Oral Mass		
CI	Calculus Index (0-3)			ONF	Oronasal Fistula		
CU	Contact Ulcer	GH	Gingival Hyperplasia	OST	Osteomyelitis	SI/E	Staining Intrinsic/Extrinsic
CR	Crowded Tooth	GI	Gingival Index (0-3)	P(mm)	Perio.Pkt. (mm)	STM	Stomatitis
DC	Dentigerous Cyst	GR	Gingival Recession	PA	Periapical Bone Lysis	SUP	Supernumerary
E	Enamel Defect	IR	Internal Resorption	ROT	Rotated Tooth	SYM/S	Symphysis Separation
EP	Epulis	LFD	Lip Fold Dermatitis	RD/R	Retained Deciduous Tooth / Root	TA/TL	Tooth Avulsion/Luxation
F	Furcation 1(v), 2(>), 3(>)	- - >	Malpositioned tooth direction			VT/NV	Vital Tooth/Nonvital
FB	Foreign Body	M	Mobile Tooth (1-3)			W	Worn Tooth

TREATMENT KEY

BE/I	Biopsy Excisional / Incisional	IL/OL	Inlay / OnLay	P&FS	Pit & Fissure Sealer	RX	Root Extraction
BFR	Buccal Fold Removal	IO	Interceptive Orthodontics	PS	Perio Surgery	VP	Vital Pulpotomy
BR	Bridge	OA/I/A/R	Orthodontic Appliance Install / Adjust / Removal	PSP	Perio Splint	WW	Wait & Watch
CM/PFM	Crown Metal/ Porcelain Fused to Metal			RA/C/I	Restoration Amalgam / Composite / Ionomer	X/XS/XSS	Extraction / Hemisect / Sx.Ext
FAR/GG/LS/RB	Apical/ FGing.Graft / Lat.Slid / Rev.Bev.	OE	Occlusal Equilibration	RC	Root Canal Trnt.		
		OI/W	Osseous Implant / Wiring	RCS	Root Canal Surgical		
FG / FV	Fluoride Gell / Varnish	OP	Odontoplasty	RPC/O	Root Planing Closed / Open		
		PC	Pulp Cap				

Occlusal Evaluation:

Oral Examination (Saliva, Breath, Tonsils, Lnn):

Periodontal Evaluation:

Gingival Index: 0 = Normal, No Swelling. 1 = No Bleeding When Probed
(GI) 2 = Bleeds When Probed 3 = Spontaneous Bleeding

Calculus Index: 0 = No Plaque 1 = Soft Film at Margin
(CI) 2 = Calculus Easily Seen 3 = Heavy Deposits

Endodontic Evaluation:

Radiographic Evaluation:

TREATMENT PLAN:

LIAISON WITH REFERRING DOCTOR

Person contacted	Phone	Record	Person

ANESTHESIA	TIME	DOSE	AGENT
Preanesthetic			
Anesth. Induct.			

E. T. size ___________GAS________
End of Procedure ________
Support ______________________________
____

PROPHYLAXIS Home Care Instructions ____________
1. Ultrasonic cleaning ____________ 2. Subgingival curettage ____________
3. Polishing ____________ 4. Other ____________

ASSESSMENT/ADDITIONAL THERAPY:

Figure 6-3 Feline Fill-in-the-Blank Dental Chart.
Courtesy of Campus Veterinary Clinic, P.C., Denver, CO.

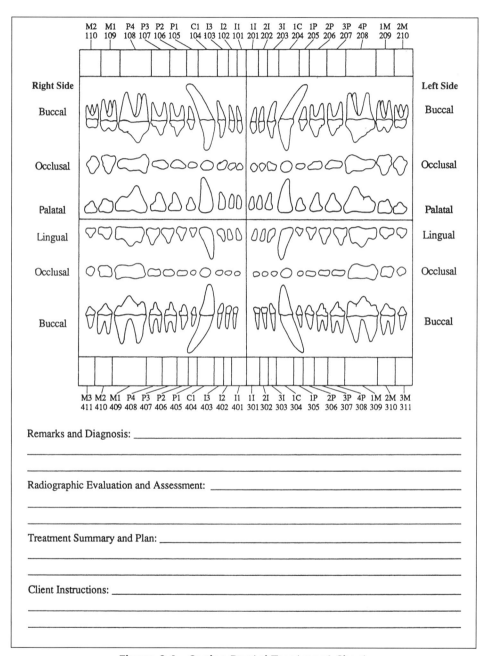

| M2 | M1 | P4 | P3 | P2 | P1 | C1 | I3 | I2 | I1 | 1I | 2I | 3I | 1C | 1P | 2P | 3P | 4P | 1M | 2M |
| 110 | 109 | 108 | 107 | 106 | 105 | 104 | 103 | 102 | 101 | 201 | 202 | 203 | 204 | 205 | 206 | 207 | 208 | 209 | 210 |

Right Side

Buccal

Occlusal

Palatal

Lingual

Occlusal

Buccal

Left Side

Buccal

Occlusal

Palatal

Lingual

Occlusal

Buccal

| M3 | M2 | M1 | P4 | P3 | P2 | P1 | C1 | I3 | I2 | I1 | 1I | 2I | 3I | 1C | 1P | 2P | 3P | 4P | 1M | 2M | 3M |
| 411 | 410 | 409 | 408 | 407 | 406 | 405 | 404 | 403 | 402 | 401 | 301 | 302 | 303 | 304 | 305 | 306 | 307 | 308 | 309 | 310 | 311 |

Remarks and Diagnosis: _____
_____
_____

Radiographic Evaluation and Assessment: _____
_____
_____

Treatment Summary and Plan: _____
_____
_____

Client Instructions: _____
_____
_____

Figure 6-4   Canine Dental Treatment Chart.
*Reprinted with permission from S. E. Holmstrom, P. Frost, and E. R. Eisner,
Veterinary Dental Techniques, 2d ed. (Philadelphia: W. B. Saunders, 1998): 13.*

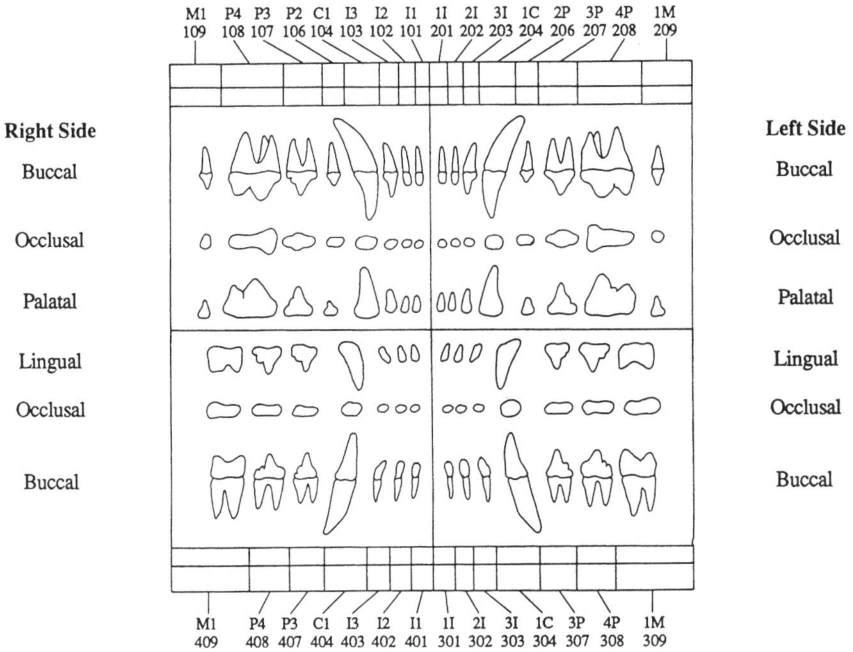

Figure 6-5   Feline Dental Treatment Chart.
Reprinted with permission from S. E. Holmstrom, P. Frost, and E. R. Eisner,
Veterinary Dental Techniques, 2d ed. (Philadelphia: W. B. Saunders, 1998): 17.

Client number _____

Pet Clinic
Initial Oral Exam

Owner _____ Patient _____ Date _____
Species _____ Breed _____ Sex _____ Date of Birth _____
Chief complaint _____
Past dental history _____
General medical history _____
Diet _____
Home oral hygiene _____
Other _____

Medical Alert

Skull type:
☐ Brachycephalic
☐ Mesocephalic
☐ Dolichocephalic
☐ _____

Oral Hygiene
☐ Plaque   N S M H
☐ Calculus   N S M H
Normal Slight Moderate Heavy

Periodontal Exam
☐ Inflammation   I C P M
☐ Gingival Edema   I C P M
☐ Pockets >3mm   I C P M
☐ Pockets >5mm   I C P M
☐ Recession   I C P M
☐ Hyperplasia   I C P M
☐ Mucogingival loss   I C P M
☐ Tooth Mobility   I C P M
☐ Further evaluation   I C P M
Incisor Canine Premolar Molar

Occlusion:
☐ Scissors
☐ Brachygnathic
☐ Prognathic
☐ Wry
☐ Level
☐ Crossbite
☐ Occlusal wear   I C P M

Tooth Abnormalities
☐ Ret. Primary   I C P
☐ Missing   I C P M
☐ Supernumerary   I C P M
☐ Caries   I C P M
☐ Resorptive   I C P M
☐ Injured   I C P M

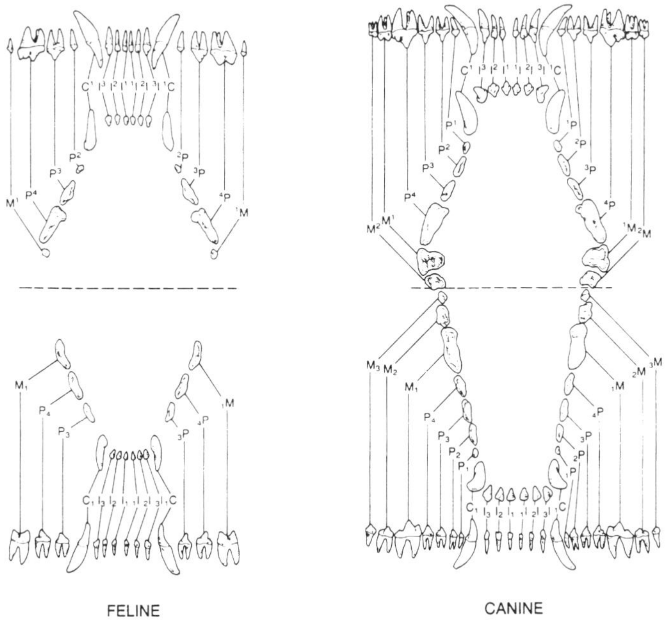

FELINE

CANINE

Figure 6-6   Pet Clinic Initial Oral Exam.
Reprinted with permission from S. E. Holmstrom, P. Frost, and E. R. Eisner,
Veterinary Dental Techniques, 2d ed. (Philadelphia: W. B. Saunders, 1998): 9.

Golden Nugget

Setting a high, low, or moderate price will position your practice in the client's mind in relation to quality.

—Robert E. Froehlich, DVM, MBA[2]

Setting Your Dental Fees

Determining the pricing strategy for your practice can be a complicated process. Understanding the costs involved in providing a service will give the practitioner a starting place for setting fees. In general, a business will be forced to close its doors if it cannot earn enough income to pay the expenses. Cost-plus pricing is a useful method to employ. Cost-plus pricing uses the formula of total fixed cost per unit + total variable cost per unit + profit margin per unit = the price or fee. The desired profit margin is the return on investment to the practice owner. Although the calculation of some costs can be arbitrary, the following process can give you a "ballpark" figure to start from when setting your fees.[3]

In Chapter 5, I began using the example of cleaning the teeth of a 60-pound dog to calculate the cost of expendables. Before calculating the fees for the dental cleaning alone, we must first determine the *total* cost to perform the service. After figuring these basic costs, we can begin to set fees so that the practice is assured of earning a profit. In Chapter 2, we calculated the overhead of the Baseline Animal Hospital. We determined that it costs Dr. Allright $1.50 per minute or $90 per hour to open the clinic doors. The basic overhead of the dental department was determined to be $9,200 per year. In Chapter 5, the basic cost of expendables for performing a 1-hour-long prophylaxis on a 60-pound dog was $18.82. As expected, the supervising veterinarian wants to earn some income from this case. If Dr. Allright's associate is the doctor, she will earn 20 percent of the production income ($108.82) or a minimum of $21.76. Dr. Allright earns approximately $33.64 per hour. Dr. Allright also budgeted $5,000 to expand dental services and purchased some new equipment for the dental department. He wants the equipment to pay for itself by earning dental production dollars. The profit from the dental department is the owner's return on investment, and Dr. Allright has set a goal of 20 percent. This amount is calculated by adding 20 percent of the subtotal cost to reach a total cost. When you perform this exercise yourself, it is a good idea to "pad" the estimate slightly by rounding up to allow for forgotten expenses, although that has not been done in this illustration. Table 6-1 illustrates these calculations.

The numbers in Table 6-1 exhibit some interesting results. The Baseline Animal Hospital must charge a minimum of $130.58 to break even. Currently, the hospital charges an average of $100 per dental case (the total of dental and anesthesia income). To improve the profitability of the hospital, the fees should be set higher

Table 6-1   The Cost of a Single Dental Cleaning

Clinic Input: Baseline Animal Hospital	Cost
Cost of expendables	$ 18.82
Overhead cost per hour (excludes veterinarian's salaries)	+ 90.00
Subtotal: minumum production income	108.82
Veterinarian's salary (20% of production income)	+ 21.76
Subtotal: cost before desired profit margin (breakeven point)	130.58
Add-on factor for profit margin (20% of subtotal)	+ 26.12
Total cost for this dental service	**$156.70**

than that amount. If Dr. Allright does nothing more than raise his fees to an average of $130 for each of his 200 dental cases, his expenses would remain the same, and gross dental income would increase by $30 per case or $6,000 per year. The entire fee increase would result in raising net income by $6,000.

It is good business practice to know the costs of your services, but it is also essential to understand the needs, wants, and perceptions of your clientele.[4] Even though Dr. Allright knows how much he needs to charge for a service, he also must know about the local demand for the service. According to David Gallagher, reporting a study done by R. K. House, veterinarians who charge higher fees tend to have higher net incomes and work shorter hours. On the other hand, veterinarians who charge lower fees are likely to have lower net incomes and work longer hours. The conclusion of the study is that it is the veterinarian's attitude toward his or her clientele that is the determining factor when setting fees. A veterinarian who sets fees lower because he or she believes the clients won't pay higher fees may be underestimating clients' willingness to pay higher fees.[5] By adding value to your services, you will be able to differentiate yourself from other practices in your area and to justify higher prices to your clients.[6] The key to success is to communicate the value of your services to your clients so that they will accept the fees that will allow the practice to grow in profitability.[7] As stated by Edward Eisner, "There is a difference between cleaning teeth and treating periodontal disease. Cleaning teeth will lead to a different message to the client and lower fees."[8]

Golden Nugget

Lumping the care of all presented oral conditions under "doing a dentistry" at one set fee is poor business at best and potentially poor medicine at worst. Evaluating each tooth on its own merit and itemizing the fees relating to individual tooth care is the best way to approach a dental case.

—Jan Bellows, All Pets Dental Clinic[9]

Creating a Dental Fee Schedule

Most veterinarians realize that the time and cost of treating a feline or small canine differs greatly from treating a giant breed canine. With that in mind, it makes little sense to charge the same fee for cleaning a cat's teeth as a Great Dane's. To allow for this difference, it is helpful to use a graduated scale of fees based on the size of the animal and the severity of the condition of the teeth. In addition to the fee for the dental service, the fees for general anesthesia should be graduated, for the same reasons. A dental prophylaxis for a three-year-old feline with a moderate amount of calculus may take 20–30 minutes from start to finish, while a six-year-old Great Dane with heavy deposits and periodontal disease may require two hours. Indeed, it is only fair to your clientele to charge each owner an appropriate fee for the services that you perform specifically for his or her pet. The owner of the cat should not subsidize the dental care of bigger dogs or dogs with more severe dental problems, nor should you undercharge the owner of the giant breed dog.

Table 6-2 is a suggested fee schedule for the Baseline Animal Hospital, with the fee for dental prophylaxis calculated as a base fee plus an increment of $.50 per minute. Remember that it costs Dr. Allright $1.50 per minute to open his doors, so the balance of the fees must be distributed over his anesthesia, examination, and hospitalization charges. This model is solely an example. A similar schedule may also be developed for anesthesia, medications, hospitalization, etc. Each practice will want to develop its own fee schedule based on its local market and circumstances particular to its own needs and practice preferences.

Calculating the total fees for a dental procedure is a process of setting the fee for each individual service with the appropriate scale or range and then adding those fees to reach a total. For advanced dental procedures such as root canal therapy, the fee should be based on the level of expertise of the practitioner performing the service, the expendables required, and the time it takes to perform the service. If you are performing the service, decide how much you believe your time is worth. Generally, a veterinarian should earn a minimum of $2–3 per minute. If a procedure takes one hour, the fee for that procedure alone should be $120 to $180, depending on the level of expertise required to perform the service. A more experienced clinician should earn a higher fee than another clinician who is less experienced. A more technically difficult procedure also warrants a higher fee.

Computer software available today allows practices to develop extensive fee schedules and to quickly produce "travel sheets" for tracking services. The dental travel sheet that Dr. Edward Eisner of the Denver Veterinary Dental Service uses is reproduced in Figure 6-7. Each dental service is shown in detail along with the other services that are involved in a dental case. For a dental specialist, these services are performed on a regular basis and this level of detail is necessary on the travel sheet. Nonspecialty practices may not wish to itemize their services in such detail. Software

Table 6-2   Baseline Animal Hospital Suggested Fee Schedule*

Species/Size of Animal	Minor Prophylaxis @ 30 Minutes	Moderate Prophylaxis @ 60 Minutes	Major Prophylaxis @ 90 Minutes
Feline	$30	$45	$60
Canine ≤ 20 lb	$35	$50	$65
Canine 21–4 0 lb	$40	$55	$70
Canine 41–80 lb	$45	$60	$75
Canine ≥ 81 lb	$50	$65	$80

* These fees do not include preoperative laboratory tests, anesthesia, radiographs, extractions, oral fluoride, or other additional therapeutic services; professional care following the procedure; or dispensed items.

packages also allow the practice to develop standard estimates for procedures done on a repeated basis and to customize the estimate for each individual patient, as seen in Figure 6-8.

Dr. Jan Bellows of the All Pets Dental Clinic in Pembroke Pines, Fla., uses the dental fee sheet in Figure 6-9. The sheet lists the fees involved in any routine or advanced dental case, beginning with the examination and including laboratory testing, anesthesia, dental fees, supportive treatment, and home care products. Dr. Bellows circles each required service with the fee and gives the client a copy to take home. The advantage of this system is that it is very quick and simple to use and does not require a computer.[10]

For more information about pricing strategies, see Robert Froehlich's series of three articles in *AAHA TRENDS Magazine* describing in greater detail the process and considerations for determining your fees.[11]

References

1. D. Erlewein and E. Kuhns, *Instructions for Veterinary Clients* (Goleta, Calif.: American Veterinary Publications, 1991): 326–327.
2. R. E. Froehlich, "Pricing Strategies for Veterinary Practices, Part I," *AAHA TRENDS Magazine* (December 1996/January 1997): 29.
3. Ibid.: 30.
4. R. E. Froehlich, "Pricing Strategies for Veterinary Practices, Part III," *AAHA TRENDS Magazine* (April/May 1997): 42.
5. D. P. Gallagher, *Business Management for the Veterinary Practitioner* (Denver, Colo.: Chubb Communications, 1995): 22–23.
6. Froehlich, "Pricing Strategies, Part I": 30.
7. R. E. Froehlich, "Pricing Strategies for Veterinary Practices, Part II," *AAHA TRENDS Magazine* (February/March 1997): 28.
8. E. R. Eisner, Personal conversations, December 1998.
9. J. Bellows, "Creating a Dental Fee Sheet," *Veterinary Forum* (July 1995): 44–46.
10. Ibid.
11. Froehlich, "Pricing Strategies for Veterinary Practices, Parts I–III."

```
Name (Last, first) _____    Client Id _____    Provider _____    Date _____

Address (Street) _____    City/State _____

New Patient? Yes  No        Patient's Name _____    Weight _____

Age _____    Breed _____    Color _____    Sex _____        Fecal? Yes  No

Reason for Appointment:
```

PHARMACY	10	___ SSAN SKIN SCRAPING AND ANALYSIS	___ IVCP INTRAVENOUS CATH PLACEMENT
		___ STT SCHIRMER TEAR TEST	___ IVSET IV ADMIN SOLUSET
___ DMEDN= DISP: (DENTAL MEDICATION)		___ UR URINALYSIS	___ IVTCON IV T-CONNECTOR
___ DPDTS= DISP:(DENTAL PRODUCTS)		___ URSC URINE SAMPLE COLLECTION	___ TATID ID TATTOO

LAB-IN HOUSE	12
___ BCBC CBC (WITH DIFFERENTIAL)	
___ BG BLOOD GLUCOSE	
___ BGOT BLOOD GLUCOSE - ONE-TOUCH	
___ BLALT BLOOD ALT TEST	
___ BLCORT CORTISOL SNAP TEST	
___ BLCR BLOOD/URINE CREATININE	
___ BLN BUN (BLOOD UREA NITROGEN)	
___ BLP12 GENERAL HEALTH PANEL 12	
___ BLP6 PRE-ANEST PANEL 6	
___ BLQBC QBC	
___ BLQBCP PRE-OP QBC	
___ BLQBPC PREOP QBC + COAGULATION	
___ BLT4 THYROID 4 SNAP	
___ BLVFLA FELINE LEUKEMIA/FIV TEST	
___ BLVFLS FELINE LEUKEMIA-SALIVA TEST	
___ BLWHW HEARTWORM TEST - DIFIL	
___ BLWHWA HEARTWORM TEST - ANTIGEN	
___ BLWHWB HEARTWORM TEST-DIFIL+ANTIGEN	
___ BSC BLOOD SAMPLE COLLECTION	
___ CY CYTOLOGY	
___ EKG ELECTROCARDIOGRAM-INITIAL	
___ EKGF ELECTROCARDIOGRAM-FOLLOW UP	
___ FDT FLUORESCEINE DYE TEST	
___ FECFLT FECAL FLOTATION TEST	
___ FECSC FECAL SAMPLE COLLECTION	
___ FEFLTD FECAL FLOTATION & DIRECT	
___ FEPROF FECAL PROFILE	
___ FLA FLUID ANALYSIS	
___ FLCY FLUID CYTOLOGY	
___ FLDCOL FLUID SAMPLE COLLECTION	
___ MICRB MICROBIOLOGY-BACTERIA	
___ MICRBF MICROBIOLOGY-BACTERIA&FUNGAL	
___ MICRF FUNGAL CULTURE	

LAB-REFERRED	13
___ BLDPRF BLOOD PROFILE	
___ BTHP BLOOD TOTAL HEALTH PROFILE	
___ CYR CYTOLOGY - REFFERED OUT	
___ HISTO HISTOPATHOLOGY	
___ MISCLR MISCELLANEOUS LAB-REFERRED	
___ THP1 THYROID PROFILE WITH PANEL	
___ THP2 THYROID3 & THYROID4	

RADIOLOGY	14
___ RA1 RADIOGRAPH - SURVEY FILMS	
___ RAA RADIOGRAPH-ADDITIONAL (EACH)	
___ RAAF RADIOGRAPH INTERPRET FEE	
___ ULTR ULTRASONOGRAPHY	
___ ULTRF ULTRASONOGRAPHY-FOLLOW UP	

HOSPITAL-HOSPITAL CARE	15
___ PCC PROFESSIONAL CARE CAT	
___ PCD PROFESSIONAL CARE DOG	
___ PCIN PROFESS CARE-INTENSIVE/DAY	
___ PCIS PROFESS CARE-ISOLATION/DAY	
___ PCPP PROF. CARE, POCKET PET	
___ SOHN1 STAY OVER,HOSP.& NOURISHMENT	
___ SOHN2 STAY OVER,HOSP.& NOURISHMENT	
___ SOHN3 STAY OVER,HOSP.& NOURISHMENT	
___ SOHN4 STAY OVER,HOSP.& NOURISHMENT	
___ SOHN5 STAY OVER,HOSP.& NOURISHMENT	

HOSPITAL-PROCEDURES	16
___ IVC INTRAVENOUS CATHETER	
___ IVCJ IV CATHETER, JUGULAR	

HOSPITAL-MEDS ADMINISTERED	17
___ ADOMH ADMIN: (ORAL MEDS) HOSP	
___ AIMH1 ADMIN: (INJECTABLE MEDS)HOSP	
___ AIMH2 ADMIN: (INJECTABLE MEDS)HOSP	
___ AIMH3 ADMIN: (INJECTABLE MEDS)HOSP	
___ AIMH4= ADMIN: (INJECTABLE MEDS)HOSP	
___ AIVF= ADMIN: (IV FLUIDS)	
___ ASCF= ADMIN: (SQ FLUIDS)	

ANESTHESIA	24
___ AEVAL PREANESTHETIC EVALUATION	
___ AEXQBC PREANESTHETIC EXAM + QBC	
___ AI1 ANESTHESIA INDUCT. FELINE	
___ AI2 ANESTHESIA INDUCT. SM DOG	
___ AI3 ANESTHESIA INDUCT. MED DOG	
___ AI4 ANESTHESIA INDUCT. LG DOG	
___ AI5 ANESTHESIA INDUCT. XL DOG	
___ AIP1 ANES.INDUCT.PROPOFOL-FELINE	
___ AIP2 ANES.INDUCT.PROPOFOL-SM.DOG	
___ AIP3 ANES.INDUCT.PROPOFOL-MED.DOG	
___ AIP4 ANES.INDUCT.PROPOFOL-LG.DOG	
___ AIP5 ANES.INDUCT.PROPOFOL-XLG.DOG	
___ AM1= ANES. ISOFLUR. MNTCE CAT	
___ AM2= ANES. ISOFLUR. MNTCE SM. DOG	
___ AM3= ANES. ISOFLUR. MNTCE MED DOG	
___ AM4= ANES. ISOFLUR. MNTCE LG. DOG	
___ AM5= ANES. ISOFLUR. MNTCE XL. DOG	
___ AMO PULSE OXIMETRY MONITORING	
___ APP ANESTHESIA POCKET PET	
___ LOAN LOCAL ANESTHESIA	
___ TRAN TRANQUILIZATION	
___ TRANBD TRANQUILIZATION-BOARDING	

```
                    ┌──────────────┐
                    │   See Back   │
                    └──────────────┘
```

Figure 6-7   Sample Dental Travel Sheet.
Courtesy of Denver Veterinary Dental Service.

```
MISC-NO CHARGE SERVICE CODES   32      ___ DLS      LATERAL SLIDING FLAP              ___ DPSREM   REMOVE PERIO. SPLINT
                                       ___ DMXFSX   MAXILLOFACIAL SURGERY             ___ DPTX     PERIODONTAL TREATMENT
___ APPT     APPOINTMENT - PLEASE SCHED ___ DSURG1   ORAL SURGERY, 1 UNIT             ___ DRPC     ROOT PLANING - CLOSED
___ CABA     CALL BACK                  ___ DSURG2   ORAL SURGERY, 2 UNITS            ___ DRPO     ROOT PLANING - SURGICAL
___ DECALL   DENTAL RECALL              ___ DSURG3   ORAL SURGERY, 3 UNITS
___ DENXT    NEXT DENTAL APPOINTMENT    ___ DSURG4   ORAL SURGERY, 4 UNITS            DENTAL-RESTORATIVE            65
___ DREM     DENTAL REMINDER            ___ DSURG=   ORAL SURGERY
                                        ___ DSURPK   DENTAL/ORAL SURGERY PACK         ___ DBLEA1   COSMETIC BLEACHING
DISCOUNTS                        47     ___ DSURPP   ORAL SURGERY, POCKET PET         ___ DBLEA2   COSMETIC BLEACHING
                                        ___ DSUT=    SUTURE PACKS                     ___ DBLEA3   COSMETIC BLEACHING
___ DIS      DISCOUNT % OF PREVIOUS ITEM ___ DW      TRANSOSSEOUS WIRING              ___ DBLEA4   COSMETIC BLEACHING
___ DISA     DISCOUNT - AMOUNT          ___ DX       TOOTH EXTN(S), ONE ROOT          ___ DBLEAC   BLEACHING SETUP
___ DISE     15% DISC.ORDER LESS DISPDS ___ DX1      LOOSE TOOTH EXTRACTION(S)        ___ DBR      DENTAL BRIDGE INSTALLED
___ DISHMP   HEALTH MAINT PLAN 10% SAVING ___ DXD    EXTRN(S). VERY DIFFICULT         ___ DFV      FLUORIDE VARNISH APPLICATION
___ DISN     10% NEW CLIENT DISCOUNT    ___ DXR      ROOT EXTRACTION(S)               ___ DOP      ODONTOPLASTY
___ DISP     PROFESSIONAL COURTESY      ___ DXS      EXTN(S)-MULTIROOT TEETH          ___ DP&FS    PIT & FISSURE SEALER
___ DISPO    DISCOUNT-PET OVERPOPULATION ___ DXSS    SURGICAL EXTRACTION(S)           ___ DRA      AMALGAM RESTORATION
                                        ___ PTUBE    PHARYNGOSTOMY TUBE               ___ DRC      COMPOSITE RESTORATION
DENTISTRY-ROUTINE                60                                                  ___ DRC2     DENTAL FILLING REPAIR
                                        DENTAL-ENDODONTICS               62          ___ DRCM     METAL CROWN
___ DPEX     DENTAL PROPHYLAXIS-EXAM ROOM                                            ___ DRCPFM   PORCELAIN CROWN
___ DPRJV    JUVENILE DENTAL CARE & FLUO ___ DAPEX   ENDO.-APEXIFICATION             ___ DREB=    RESTORATION-ENAMEL BONDING
___ DPRMI1   DENT.PROPHYLAXIS MINOR CAT ___ DPC      ENDODONTICS-PULP CAP             ___ DRI1     1ST GL.IONOMER FILLING
___ DPRMI2   DENT.PROPHYLAXIS MINOR SMDOG ___ DRC1D  ROOT CANAL TMT. DOG INCISOR     ___ DRI2     ADDIT. GL.ION. FILLING(S)
___ DPRMI3   DENT.PROPHYLAXIS MINOR MDDOG ___ DRC2D  ROOT CANAL TMT. DOG CANINE      ___ DRIL     RESTORATIVE INLAY
___ DPRMI4   DENT.PROPHYLAXIS MINOR LGDOG ___ DRC3D  ROOT CANAL TMT. DOG UPPER P4    ___ DRIMP    IMPRESSIONS FOR RESTORATION
___ DPRMI5   DENT.PROPHYLAXIS MINOR XLDOG ___ DRC4D  ROOT CANAL TMT. DOG LOWER M1    ___ DROL     RESTORATIVE ONLAY
___ DPRMO1   DENT.PROPHYLAXIS MOD. CAT  ___ DRC5D    ROOT CANAL DOG 2ROOTED TOOTH    ___ DROTH=   RESTORATIVE DENTISTRY
___ DPRMO2   DENT.PROPHYLAXIS MOD.SM. DOG ___ DRC6D  ROOT CANAL TMT. DOG UPPER M1    ___ DRPB=    RESTORATION-PREP/BUILDUP
___ DPRMO3   DENT.PROPHYLAXIS MOD.MED.DOG ___ DRC7F  ROOT CANAL TMT. FEL. INCISOR
___ DPRMO4   DENT.PROPHYLAXIS MOD.LG. DOG ___ DRC8F  ROOT CANAL TMT.FELINE CANINE    Additional Services:
___ DPRMO5   DENT.PROPHYLAXIS MOD.XL. DOG ___ DRC9F  ROOT CANAL TMT. FEL. P4 / M1
___ DPRMX1   DENT.PROPHYLAXIS MAJOR CAT ___ DRCPP    ROOT CANAL TMT. POCKET PET      _____
___ DPRMX2   DENT.PROPHYLAXIS MAJ.SM. DOG ___ DRCS   SURG. ROOT CANAL TMT            _____
___ DPRMX3   DENT.PROPHYLAXIS MAJ.MED. DOG ___ DSUP  DENTAL SUPPLIES                 _____
___ DPRMX4   DENT.PROPHYLAXIS MAJ.LG. DOG ___ DVP    VITAL PULPOTOMY                 _____
___ DPRMX5   DENT.PROPHYLAXIS MAJ.XL. DOG                                            _____
___ DRAD     DENTAL RADIOGRAPHS-SURVEY  DENTAL-ORTHODONTICS              63          _____
___ DRAD2    ADDITIONAL SURVEY X-RAYS                                               _____
___ DRCONS   DENTAL XRAY CONSULTATION   ___ DAA      ORTHODONTIC ADJUSTMENT          _____
___ DRDIO1   1ST INTRAORAL X-RAY        ___ DAI      INSTALL ORTHO. APPLIANCE        Dispensed Medications:
___ DRDIO2   ADDITIONAL INDIVIDUAL X-RAYS ___ DAR    ORTHO. APPLIANCE REMOVAL
___ DRDUP    DUPLICATE 1 DENTAL X-RAY   ___ DDIR=    ORTHODONTICS-DIRECT             _____
___ DRDUP2   DUPLICATE SET, DENTAL XRAYS ___ DELB=   ORTHODONTICS-ELASTICS/BRACKT    _____
___ DSPHOT   DENTAL STUDY PHOTOGRAPHS   ___ DIMP     ORTHODONTICS-IMPRESSIONS        _____
                                        ___ DIO      INTERCEPTIVE ORTHODONTICS       _____
DENTISTRY-SURGERY                61     ___ DOE      OCCLUSAL EQUILIBRATION          _____
                                                                                    _____
___ DBFR     SURG. BUCCAL FOLD REMOVAL  DENTAL-PERIODONTICS              64          _____
___ DBIOPE   ORAL BIOPSY, EXCISIONAL                                                _____
___ DBIOPI   ORAL BIOPSY - INCISIONAL   ___ DFG      FLOURIDE TREATMENT              Notes:
___ DFAR     APICAL REPOSITION FLAP     ___ DORTX    ORAL MEDICAL THERAPY
___ DFGG     FREE GINGIVAL GRAFT        ___ DPP      PERIODONTAL PACKING             _____
___ DFLS     GINGIVAL SLIDING FLAP SURG. ___ DPRCHX  DEEP ROOT THERAPY              _____
___ DFRB     REVERSE BEVEL FLAP SURG.   ___ DPS      PERIODONTAL SURGERY             _____
___ DGY      SURGICAL GINGIVECTOMY      ___ DPSCHX   SUBGINGIVAL MEDICAL THERAPY    _____
___ DI       OSSEOUS IMPLANT            ___ DPSP     PERIODONTAL SPLINT             _____
```

Figure 6-7 (*continued*)   Sample Dental Travel Sheet.

```
                    CAMPUS VETERINARY CLINIC, P.C.
                     2186 S. Colorado Blvd., Suite C
                            Denver, CO 80222
                  Phone 303-757-8481  Fax 303-759-4729


                         *** Estimate ***
_____

  Client: 400           Animal: ROCKY          Date: 12/31/98
          EDWARD R EISNER
  Notes.: SAMPLE ESTIMATE-ROUTINE PROPHYLAXIS    Number: 0003764
_____


   PREANESTHETIC EVALUATION           1.00   $00.00 -     $00.00
   ANESTHESIA INDUCT. LG DOG          1.00    00.00 -      00.00
   ANES. ISOFLUR. MNTCE LG. DOG       1.00    00.00 -      00.00
   PULSE OXIMETRY MONITORING          1.00    00.00 -      00.00
   DENT.PROPHYLAXIS MOD.LG. DOG       1.00    00.00 -      00.00
   PROFESSIONAL CARE DOG              1.00    00.00 -      00.00
   Additionally, X-rays, dental treatment and extractions
   will be performed if indicated.
                                             ---------------------
                           Estimated Total:   $00.00 -     $00.00
_____


   HOSPITAL POLICY:      (COPY OF ESTIMATE GIVEN TO OWNER Y / N)
   This is only an estimate of services.  We want to try to give you the
   best possible care for your special companion.  In order to do so,

   occasionally the anesthetic or procedure time will be increased.  Also,
   we sometimes must run tests or do procedures that we did not anticipate
   when giving you this estimate.  We will do our very best to inform you
   of any tests or procedures we must do which will cause an increase in
   this estimate figure.  Our job is to give your pet the best possible
   medical and surgical care available at a reasonable cost to both of
   us.

   ABANDONMENT:
   If the patient is not removed, written notice will be mailed five (5) day

   after the proposed release date, to the last known address, to remove the
   animal.  If the patient is not removed from this hospital within seven (7

   days of such mailing, said animal will be considered abandoned and may be
   disposed of or euthanized.  I understand that abandonment of the animal
   does not relieve the owner or the undersigned of the financial obligation
   for services rendered.

   RISK:
   I understand, as with any procedure or anesthetic, there are certain
   risks. The expected chance of survival for the above described procedure
   is (poor/fair/good/very good/excellent).  Some nonfatal complications, not
   mentioned above, which have been seen other than self inflicted trauma or
   too much exercise are:_____
```

Figure 6-8   Computer-Generated Standard Estimate.
Courtesy of Campus Veterinary Clinic, P.C., Denver, CO.

```
  EDWARD R EISNER                        Number: 0003764  Page: 2
```
===

even when proper care is administered after release from the hospital. I
understand that normally complications are relatively minor and can be
corrected without difficulty. However, I have been advised that certain
complications are serious and may necessitate further treatment and
expenses. I understand that an attendant is not on the hospital premises
24 hours per day and that after hours care is provided as necessary in the
judgement of the veterinarians in charge.

EXTENT OF SERVICE DESIRED:
Should unforseen, nonemergency procedures not listed above be necessary
and desirable in the attending veterinarian's professional judgement:
_____ I prefer Campus Veterinary Clinic to proceed with all procedures.
_____ I prefer to be telephoned prior to any additional procedures, other
        than emergencies. However, if I cannot be reached, I authorize
        unforeseen, nonemergency procedures.
_____ If I cannot be reached, I do not authorize unforeseen nonemergency
        procedures.

AUTHORIZATION TO TREAT:
The undersigned certifies that s/he is the owner of and/or the responsibl
person for the animal described above and gives permission for the

treatment(s) described:_____

(with/without anesthesia/sedation) as necessary. I understand that the
procedure necessitating the procedure(s) is:_____
and that this treatment as well as alternative forms of treatment have
been explained to me.

QUOTES ON PROPOSED SERVICES ARE VALID FOR 60 DAYS.

Phone numbers where I can be reached today:

_____
        Home   Work   Other

PAYMENT WILL BE:

_____ Cash   If payment, as quoted above, cannot be mad
_____ Check   in full at the time of service, payment ar-
_____ Complete Care   rangements must be made prior to treatment.
_____ Discover   A monthly service charge of 1.5% or a minimum
_____ Mastercard   of $3.00 is applied to all balances. The per
_____ Visa   son responsible for this animal will be re-
_____ American Express   responsible for all attorney fees and collect
                                costs should steps be necessary.

Signature_____ Date____/____/____

Figure 6-8 (*continued*)   Computer-Generated Standard Estimate.

All Pets Dental Clinic
9111 Taft Street
Pembroke Pines, Florida 33024
Phone: (954) 432-1111 Fax: (954) 431-8550

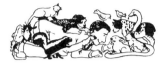

FEES FOR DENTAL CLINIC
1998

Dental Consultation	Exam	DEX
Preoperative Testing	Complete Blood Count	CBC
<1 YR CB , EKG Heartcheck	Kidney Function Test	KFT
1-7 YRS CBC, TOTAL PROTEIN	Liver Function Test	LFT
LIVER, KIDNEY, GLUCOSE,	Total Protein Test	TPT
COAGULATION, EKG Heartcheck	Glucose	BST
>7 YRS CBC, ORGAN PROFILE,	Chest X-Ray	XRCH
ELECTROLYTES, URINE, EKG,	Organ Profile	CPT
CHEST X-RAY, COAGULATION	Electrolytes	ELEC
	Coagulation Profile	COAG
	Complete Urinalysis	UAC
	EKG Heartcheck	ECGS
	Intravenous Catheter	SETIV
	Intravenous Fluids	FLUID
Pre-Anesthetic Sedation	. . . .	MSED
Local Anesthesia (Per Quadrant)	. . . .	LOCAL
Anesthesia per hour	. . . .	ANES
Anes Monitoring/Telemetry	. . . .	POX
Dental Radiographs	One to Three Views	DRAD
	Each Additional View	DRADA
Cleaning and Polishing	Gingivitis	DCPG
	Advanced Gingivitis	DCPGA
	Periodontics	DCPP
	Flouride Treatment	DFL
Endodontics	Single Rooted Tooth	DEND1
	Double Rooted Tooth	DEND2
	Triple Rooted Tooth	DEND3
	Surgical Endodontics - Apicoectomy	DENDS
Extractions	Single Rooted Tooth (first premolar, incisor)	DEXT1
	Double Rooted Tooth	DEXT2
	Triple Rooted Tooth	DEXT3
	Canine	DEXTC
	Deciduous Tooth	DEXTD
Crowns	Rubber Impressions	DCRI
	Crown Prep	DCP
	Lab Fees	DCLF
	Crown Cementation	DCC
	Post Crown Medication	PCMED
	Repeat Anesthesia and Pulse Oximeter	DCRA
Periodontics	Flap Surgery (per quadrant)	DPFS
	Root Planing	DPRP
	Gingivectomy	DPG
	Perioceutical	PERC
	Guided Tissue Regeneration	DPGTR
Restorative Care	Cat Neck Lesion - Glass Ionomer	DRNL
	Bonding	DRB
Orthodontics	Stone Study Models	DOSS
	Orthodontic Care	DOC
	Lab Fees	DOLF
	Sterile Extraction Pack	SEP
	Sterile Perio Pack	SPP
	Laser Unit Fee	LASR
Antibiotic Injection	. . . .	IANT
Discomfort Injection	. . . .	IP
Hospitalization	Per Night	HOSP
Home Care	Antibiotic (ANL - AN25 - AN75 - A150)	
	Pain Relief Medication (RM25 - RM100)	

Figure 6-9   Dental Fee Sheet.
Courtesy of All Pets Dental Clinic, Pembroke Pines, FL.

CHAPTER 7

Marketing Your Dental Services

> **Golden Nugget**
>
> Marketing is a social and managerial process by which individuals and groups obtain what they need and want through creating, offering, and exchanging products of value with others.
>
> —Philip Kotler [1]

Your dental program is in place. You have attended seminars, purchased equipment, and prepared your dental records and fee schedules. It is time to perform dentistry. The next phase of developing your profitable dental department is to begin to market your services. Your current client base is your greatest asset and the best place to start. Your clients are already familiar with your practice, and they come to your office because they trust you. It is much easier to promote your services to the clients that you already have than it is to find new clients and enroll them with the dental emphasis.

Marketing is a dirty word to some people. When we think of marketing, car salespeople and telemarketers come to mind. Marketing doesn't need to be a negative concept. Without realizing it, you engage in marketing practices every day when you offer your treatment recommendations to your clients and ask them to schedule an appointment. You engage in marketing when you send reminders and newsletters and engage in other routine practice activities. Marketing a service that you believe in can be an enjoyable activity.

Traditionally, business course instructors identify the classic components of marketing as the four "Ps": product (dentistry), place (in your hospital or materials from your practice), price (fees, discussed in Chapter 6), and promotion. In addition, there are three types of marketing: internal, interactive, and external.

▲ *Internal marketing* is the effort within a company to train and motivate its client-contact employees and support staff to work as a team to provide client satisfaction.

▲ *Interactive marketing* describes the staff's skill in handling customer contact. As Philip Kotler states in *Marketing Management:*

> In services marketing, the service quality is enmeshed with the service delivery. This is especially true of professional services. The client judges service quality not only by its *technical quality* (e.g., Was the surgery successful?) but also by its functional quality (e.g., Did the surgeon show concern and inspire confidence?). Professionals cannot assume that they will satisfy the patient simply because they provide good technical service. Therefore, the professional has to master the skills of interactive marketing.[2]

▲ *External marketing* describes the normal activities of a business performed to service its existing and new customers.[3] Your clientele is familiar with you and your staff. The pet owners look to you for advice about the care of their pets, which they value as family members. The cost of marketing to your own clients is relatively inexpensive. External marketing also describes efforts to attract new customers to your business and to educate them about the services and philosophy of your practice. It is much more expensive to seek new clients. While it is important to maintain a constant flow of new clients to replace departing clients and to allow the practice to grow, your current clientele is an audience ready to listen and act. In this chapter, I present tools for marketing dental services to your clients (interactive and external marketing). There are many different ideas and techniques; you should choose the ideas that work the best for you.

The Veterinary Dental Team

The target group for internal marketing is your own staff. If your staff isn't part of your dental marketing effort, you probably won't have a significant dental program. Your first task is to teach them the importance of regular dental care for companion animals so that they come to share the same beliefs. Your receptionists and technicians are your best assets in client communications and interactive marketing. With proper training, education, and inspiration, your entire staff will become partners in building a growing dental practice.

Receptionists

Your receptionists have the first and last contacts with your clients. They answer the telephone and schedule the appointments. A good reception team will review the patient's records before the visit and be prepared to recommend needed services, such as dental care. At the end of each visit, the team will reinforce your treatment philosophy, collect the fees, and schedule the next appointment or advise the client when to expect the next reminder for dental care.

Technicians
The veterinary technicians are invaluable in a dental practice because they allow the veterinarian to delegate much of the dental care and thereby increase clinic productivity. Technicians are trained to perform the tasks described in Chapter 4. During a prophylaxis, a well-trained technician can uncover conditions that require advanced dentistry, such as root canal therapy for a fractured carnassial tooth that is obscured by calculus. Technicians enhance the perceived value of the service when they telephone clients after the procedure to inform them of the animal's postoperative recovery and the success of the treatment. Technicians may also be skilled at giving discharge instructions and teaching home care.

Hospital Assistants and Kennel Staff
By assisting the veterinarians and technicians, these staff members can aid the practice in building the dental department.

Tools for Interactive Marketing During the Office Visit
There are many areas of opportunity for marketing dental services during your regular practice activities.

The Physical Examination
The physical exam is the key to the success of your action plan (see Chapter 3). Use every physical examination as an opportunity to examine the oral cavity. Even if the client is visiting for a different reason, it only takes a second to lift the lips and look for signs of dental pathology. Each visit should be used to educate the client on the importance of regular dental care for the long-term well-being of the pet.

When you discover a condition that requires dental treatment, show the client what you observe. Point out the redness and swelling of the gums, use a periodontal probe to point out pus pockets and exposed roots. If the patient has plaque, tartar, or halitosis, explain to the client the risk of bacteria infecting the bloodstream and organs. Most clients will want to help their pets once they are aware of a problem.[4]

A client should never leave your office without the benefit of the Rule of 3Rs. Plan a phone call to check your patient's well-being, schedule a recheck appointment, or set up a reminder for the next time services are due.

Photography
Use photographs as a client information tool. Polaroid and digital cameras take instant pictures that you can use to educate your clients about dental care and to show them the seriousness of their pets' dental problems.[5] A picture is worth a thousand words. It is your job to convince the pet owner that there is a problem and the

pet's health is at stake. One advantage of a photograph is that it can illustrate a painful problem without hurting the pet and can reduce the risk of injury to both client and staff members if the patient is unpredictable or fractious. You can also give the client the photograph to take home to help convince other family members.

Smile Book

Document your dental cases with photographs and build a portfolio of before-and-after cases. An album of photos of dental procedures performed in the hospital can be a very useful aid in describing dental care and gaining compliance. Pharmacia and Upjohn (Kalamazoo, Michigan; see Appendix C for complete address) has produced two Smile Books, one on dental pathology and the other on dental radiography. These books feature color photographs with easy-to-understand captions that illustrate the benefits of dental treatment. They are available at no charge to use for client education.

Bulletin Board

Use a bulletin board to highlight dental care at your office. You can feature a dental success story and display before-and-after photographs of happy pets and their owners.

Brochures

The AAHA and other professional associations have produced dental care brochures to use as client education tools for their members. Also, companies in the dental industry publish brochures that promote dental care and their products. These brochures are professionally prepared, use high-quality graphic art and color photographs, and are written for easy understanding. Most veterinarians lack the resources to produce comparable materials. The companies that produce home care products (for example, Addison Biological Laboratory, Hill's Pet Nutrition, Pharmacia and Upjohn, and VRx Pharmaceuticals; see Appendix C for complete addresses) have produced some of the best brochures.

Home Care Instructions and Handouts

There are times when professionally prepared brochures do not communicate everything that you want your clients to know. You may wish to develop some home care instructions (see Figures 7-1 and 7-2) or written information to give to your clients. Use a desktop publishing program or the services of a printer to produce attractive materials on colored paper.

Client Education Aids: Models and Posters

A number of models and posters are available for client education. Anatomically correct models of the canine and feline oral dentition with healthy and pathological displays are useful for demonstrating the common oral diseases. You can use a model to show the client the difference between a normal mouth and the condition observed in the pet's mouth. Both naturally colored and clear models are available

EDWARD R. EISNER, D.V.M.
Diplomate, American Veterinary Dental College
PHILLIP W. CARLSON, D.V.M.

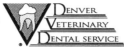

DENVER VETERINARY DENTAL SERVICE

CAMPUS VETERINARY CLINIC, P.C.
2186 South Colorado Boulevard, Suite C
Denver, Colorado 80222
Phone (303) 757-8481
FAX (303) 759-4729

HOME DENTAL CARE FOLLOWUP RECOMMENDATIONS FOR DOGS

_____ on _____ has received dental treatment today. Included in the therapy was a thorough teeth cleaning, subgingival planing, and polishing to reduce the recurrence of further tartar buildup. By following the guidelines below you will be able, at home, to dramatically help your pet's teeth to remain clean and healthy longer.

ADDITIONAL THERAPY PERFORMED:

AREAS TREATED AND NEEDING
PARTICULAR ATTENTION

PROGNOSIS:
It is not unusual to see blood tinged drinking water 1-2 days after receiving dental care.

FEEDING INSTRUCTIONS:
Eating soon after recovering from a general anesthetic can produce nausea.
Tonight please offer only _____ cup solid food and _____ cup of water after _____:00 pm. If there is no digestive problem, the same amount can be offered 1 hour later.

MEDICATIONS & HOME CARE:
Animals are not fully coordinated after awakening from general anesthesia.
To prevent injury, please monitor your pet until coordination returns.

RECOMMENDED FOLLOWUP APPOINTMENTS:

RECOMMENDATIONS FOR HOME DENTAL CARE: The more you can help, the less we have to help.

- The first step in achieving quality home care for your dog is to make the therapy a pleasant experience. If there is a battle surely you will lose. Begin Slowly! Simply lift his or her lip and touch the teeth and gums for several days to familiarize your dog with having its mouth handled.

- Next, progress to rubbing the teeth and gums with your finger. As your dog accepts your attentions, wrap a small cloth or gauze around your finger and continue to rub the teeth and gums. It is best to use a pet dentifrice (sold here) and dab the moistened material into the dentifrice before rubbing the teeth. Most dogs dislike human toothpastes as they often contain detergents which foam and frighten your pet.

- Concentrate on the outside surface of the teeth as the tongue will collect excess dentifrice and the dog will itself cleanse the inside surface of the teeth.

- It is best, if your dog will permit, to use a soft tooth brush as it will more efficiently remove packed food and soft plaque from the vulnerable crevice that lies between the teeth and the gums. This crevice is the actual site of periodontal damage and infection. Move the brush back and forth along the gumline. The back teeth and the fangs are very important areas as these are places where saliva and plaque accumulate.

- Brushing three times a week is usually sufficient although with periodontal disease brushing daily can make the difference between saving and losing teeth.

The above care will greatly improve your pets dental health and lessen the frequency needed for professional dental care.

THANK YOU FOR LETTING US HELP MAINTAIN YOUR PET'S DENTAL HEALTH.

Figure 7-1   Home Dental Care Instructions for Dogs.
Courtesy of Campus Veterinary Clinic, P.C., Denver, CO.

EDWARD R. EISNER, D.V.M.
Diplomate, Amer. Vet. Dental College
Campus Veterinary Clinic, P.C.
2186 South Colorado Boulevard, Suite C
Denver, Colorado 80222
Phone (303) 757-8481 FAX (303) 759-4729

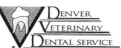
DENVER
VETERINARY
DENTAL SERVICE

CAMPUS VETERINARY CLINIC, P.C.

FELINE

HOME DENTAL CARE FOLLOWUP RECOMMENDATIONS FOR CATS

_____ on _____ has received dental treatment today. Included in the therapy was a thorough teeth cleaning, subgingival planing, and polishing to reduce the recurrence of further tartar buildup. By following the guidelines below you will be able, at home, to dramatically help your pet's teeth to remain clean and healthy longer.

ADDITIONAL THERAPY PERFORMED:

AREAS TREATED AND
NEEDING PARTICULAR ATTENTION

PROGNOSIS:

It is not unusual to see blood tinged drinking water 1-2 days after receiving dental care.

FEEDING INSTRUCTIONS:
Eating soon after recovering from general anesthetic can produce nausea. Tonight please offer only _____ tablespoons solid food and _____ ounces of water after _____:00 p.m.
If there is no digestive problem, the same amount can be offered one (1) hour later.

MEDICATIONS & HOME CARE:
Animals are not fully coordinated after awakening from general anesthesia. To prevent injury, please monitor your pet until coordination returns.

RECOMMENDED FOLLOWUP APPOINTMENTS:

RECOMMENDATIONS FOR HOME DENTAL CARE: The more you can help the less we have to help.

- The first step in achieving quality home care for your cat is to make the therapy a pleasant experience. If there is a battle surely you will lose. Begin Slowly! Simply lift his or her lip and touch the teeth and gums for several days to familiarize your cat with having its mouth handled.

- Next, progress to rubbing the teeth and gums with your finger. As your cat accepts your attentions, wrap a small cloth or gauze around your finger and continue to rub the teeth and gums. It is best to use a pet dentifrice (sold here) and dab the moistened material into the dentifrice before rubbing the teeth. Most cats dislike human toothpastes as they often contain detergents which foam and frighten your pet.

- Concentrate on the outside surface of the teeth as the rough tongue will collect excess dentifrice and the cat will itself cleanse the inside surface of the teeth.

- It is best, if your cat will permit, to use a small soft tooth brush as it will more efficiently remove packed food and soft plaque from the vulnerable crevice that lies between the teeth and the gums. This crevice is the actual site of periodontal damage. Move the brush back and forth along the gumline. The back teeth and the fangs are very important areas as these are places where saliva and plaque accumulate.

- Brushing two or three times a week is usually sufficient although with advanced periodontal disease brushing daily can make the difference between saving and losing teeth.

The above care will greatly improve your pet's dental health and lessen the frequency needed for professional dental prophylaxis.

THANK YOU FOR LETTING US HELP MAINTAIN YOUR PET'S DENTAL HEALTH.

DVDS 7

Figure 7-2   Home Dental Care Instructions for Cats.
Courtesy of Campus Veterinary Clinic, P.C., Denver, CO.

from suppliers such as Henry Schein, Inc., Pharmacia and Upjohn, Butler Company, and Dr. Shipp's Laboratories (see Appendix C for addresses). VRx Pharmaceuticals has produced an exceptionally well-done, laminated poster for client education that illustrates the various stages of gingivitis. While pathology posters are educational, clients do not appreciate being shocked by graphic photos. Pharmacia and Upjohn has also distributed a spiral flip-book of the progression of dental disease, with beautifully drawn artwork and an appealing dog as the "star." They also have produced a set of color transparencies of canine and feline gingivitis that can be displayed on an X-ray viewbox.

Videotapes

A number of videotapes are available for client education. Pharmacia and Upjohn has produced a series of three client education videotapes on dental prophylaxis, endodontics, and periodontal disease.[6] Other manufacturers in the dental field have produced tapes as well.

Intraoral Videography and Photography

Human dentists have been using intraoral cameras for years with great success. The dentist or veterinarian can use the camera for educational and marketing purposes. Digital and SLR cameras with a macro-lens can be used for intraoral close-up images of the oral cavity. The MedRx Video Vetscope (MedRx Inc™, Seminole, Fla.; see Appendix C for address) is an endoscope and intraoral camera that can be used as a marketing tool or surgical endoscope; it costs approximately $9,000.

Golden Nugget

The 3Rs are Recall–Recheck–Reminder. The Rule of 3Rs states that every client visit should end with at least one of the 3Rs as the next planned contact.

Tools for External Marketing Between Client Visits

There are a number of ways in which you can market to your clients outside the clinic.

Newsletters

Promotions for "Dental Health Months" through the clinic newsletter can be a very successful marketing tool for increasing awareness of dental issues. Use the newsletter to explain the importance of dental care to the health of the animal and offer an incentive to have the service performed. A free dental exam and discount on services annually or biannually can quickly help build a dental practice. If your practice routinely experiences slow months, use dental promotions to increase production income in those months. A partnership among the dental associations and Hill's Pet Nutrition has sponsored National Pet Dental Health Month annually in February.

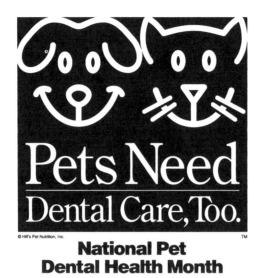

Figure 7-3   National Pet Dental Health Month Logo.
Courtesy of Hill's Pet Nutrition.

Promotional materials are available to veterinarians and may be downloaded from Hill's Web site, *www.petdental.com.* The promotional packages include camera-ready articles and artwork along with the highly identifiable logo (see Figure 7-3). Remember to conclude your dental article with a "call to action" and your phone number.

Recall Telephone Contact

Have your receptionist or technician telephone your client between 24 and 72 hours after the dental treatment to follow up on the status of your patient. The caller can answer questions your client might have about either anesthetic recovery or the dental procedure and clarify instructions. By showing your concern for the animal, you will favorably impress your clients.

Recheck Appointments

Follow-up recheck appointments allow you to track the progress of your patient and make adjustments in the treatment plan, if necessary. For more complicated cases, you can assure yourself and your client that the patient is healing well. This is an opportunity to answer questions, clarify instructions, and reinforce the need for the dental treatment. The appropriate interval for scheduling a recheck appointment might be two weeks following extractions or one month after giving home care instructions for brushing. Ask your client for feedback about his or her satisfaction with your services. By showing your client that you are concerned about the pet, you will gain esteem in your client's eyes. The best marketing tool is good word-of-mouth. When you exceed your clients' expectations, they will refer their friends and family to your practice.

Reminders

A computerized reminder system will facilitate the generation of reminders for a dental examination. Dental reminders may be included with all the other services for which an animal is due. It is also possible to send a special reminder for dental services only. At our office, we send reminders for *dental examinations* rather than *dental cleanings* because we are concerned that the anticipation of the expense of a cleaning may deter some clients from bringing in their pets. During the examination, you may find that a pet owner has been providing excellent home care and may be able to postpone the pet's next anticipated dental cleaning. A number of reminder cards have been developed especially for dental services; they feature appealing drawings or photographs of dogs and cats. Cards are available preprinted with a dental message or left blank for you to insert your own text. If you don't have a computer system, your staff may prepare reminder cards by hand. In this case, they should prepare the reminder cards at the conclusion of each visit and store them in a card file for future mailing. By using this technique, reminders are less likely to be overlooked. Sources for reminder cards are listed in Table 7-1.

National Promotions

Take advantage of national dental promotions such as the National Pet Dental Health Month. In the past, Hill's Pet Nutrition has staged art and photographic contests for children and a dental promotion contest for veterinarians. It is economically efficient to coordinate your hospital's dental health programs with the television, radio, and print media programs of the allied dental industries. VRx, manufacturer of home dental care products, also coordinates its dental promotions with National Pet Dental Health Month.

Table 7-1   Sources for Reminder Cards and Promotional Products

Supplier	Address	Telephone Number
Barx Bros.	Athens, GA	800-344-6004
Eldorado Arts	Boulder, CO	800-248-2820
Fine Line Collection	Bend, OR	800-285-1657
Histacount–Veterinary	Thorofare, NJ	800-645-5220
Idexx Informatics	Effingham, IL	888-224-4408
MBS Communications	Altamont, IL	800-887-4877
Medical Arts Press	Minneapolis, MN	800-328-0023
Sharper Cards	San Francisco, CA	800-561-6677
Smart Practice	Phoenix, AZ	800-522-0800
Sole Source	Bend, OR	800-285-1657
Straight Status	New Castle, IN	800-428-8855
The Ultra Group	Amherst, NY	800-265-2644
United Ad Label (UAL)	Brea, CA	800-423-4643
Vet Source	Rochester, NY	800-241-9324
We Create	Bend, OR	800-736-1458

Tools for External Marketing to Attract New Clients

External marketing to attract new clients is best attempted after your dental health program is well established and successful. It involves making greater efforts to reach potential new clients and educate them about the benefits of dental care. You have to sell yourself and your ideas. These external marketing techniques tend to be more costly, with less benefit. The response rate is typically much lower (less than 1–2 percent is normal) than the response you will observe with your established clientele. Following is a brief list of possibilities for external marketing.

1. **Schools and animal shelters:** Volunteer to speak at local schools and shelters about pet care and include the importance of dental care. Hand out clinic brochures, business cards, client education materials, free samples, and balloons to focus attention on you and your hospital. Offer free examinations for new adoptions to attract potential new clients to your practice.

2. **Breed clubs and obedience classes:** Give presentations to obedience classes and dog and cat breed clubs. Distribute brochures, handouts, business cards, and free samples.

3. **Dog and cat shows:** Volunteer to represent your local veterinary association at the local shows during National Pet Dental Health Month.

4. **Veterinary associations:** List your name on the local and state association speaker list. This will create opportunities to meet potential clients as well as to re-emphasize your visibility and community spirit to your established clients.

5. **Mailing lists:** Purchase bar-coded zip code mailing lists and send offers and promotions to people living in your local zip codes. It is economical to purchase a bulk rate permit from the Postal Service for bulk mailings. You can save substantial amounts of postage money, especially when using bar-coded labels. The mailing instructions are not difficult to learn, and postal workers are available at bulk mailing units to explain regulations.

6. **Coupon programs:** Offer dental care through bulk mail advertising companies such as Money Mailer, Val-Pak, or local coupon vendors. These programs are fairly economical considering the large quantity of addresses reached, but the response rate is typically only 1–2 percent. This type of program is more useful when a practice is new and trying to gain some exposure in the community.

References

1. P. Kotler, *Marketing Management* (Englewood Cliffs, N.J.: Prentice Hall, Inc., 1991): 4.
2. Ibid.: 460.
3. Ibid.: 459–460.
4. S. C. Fisher, "Associates in Practice: Production Reports Provide Great Feedback," *DVM Newsmagazine* (December 1998): 46.
5. S. E. Holmstrom, "Cameras and Computers in Dentistry," in *Proceedings of Veterinary Dentistry '98 of the 12th Annual Veterinary Dental Forum,* New Orleans, (Office of the Veterinarian Dental Association, Nashville, Tenn. 1998): 265.
6. J. Bellows, Fox News "Pet News." Courtesy of Pharmacia and Upjohn, April 12, 1997: three videotapes: *Fractured Teeth* (V-77256-A), *Periodontal Disease* (V-77256-B), *Feline Dental Care* (V-77256-C).

CHAPTER 8

Putting It All Together

Golden Nugget

Performing high-quality dental care is the key to building a successful dental department.

Perform the Service

You are ready to perform dental services. You and your staff have attended continuing education conferences, and your equipment is installed and ready to use. You published a newsletter focused on the importance of dental care, and you have mailed reminders to your target group of clients. It is time to start tracking the success of your new marketing program.

The techniques for performing dental services are beyond the scope of this book. Chapter 4 contains lists of educational opportunities and references for the medical aspects of performing dental services. The first golden nugget of this chapter states the first key to building a successful dental department. The other key is believing that what you are offering is the best health care possible for your patients. Satisfied clients with pets that are thriving, living longer, and enjoying a high quality of life are the best reward for a practitioner. The true test of success is clients who are so pleased with your services that they refer their family and friends to you. Your practice will grow as a result.

The following are a few few points about the actual services that are often overlooked but are important from the standpoint of patient and staff safety and client perception.

Communication

The importance of communication cannot be overstated. The visit with your client is an opportunity for you to educate that person about the benefits of dental care and to fully explain the treatment plan and your fees. Allow time for the client to ask questions and remember to listen to his or her concerns. Most clients are concerned about the risk of anesthesia and the cost of the procedure. Explain your anesthesia protocol and the steps you take to ensure the safety of the pet. Use fee estimates from your computer system or a fee schedule similar to the schedule illustrated in Figure 6-9 (p. 72). It is important to communicate clearly to the client your treatment plan and the costs to prevent misunderstandings when the pet is ready for release. Whether you present the estimate or a staff member does, an informed client is more likely to be a satisfied client. Clients can accept failure but hate surprises.[1]

High-Quality Service

Dental care should be performed with a high level of quality. Make it your clinic's goal to perform the best dental care possible and communicate this goal to your clients. Training and experience are required to provide service at the highest level.

Patient Safety

Anesthetic intubation and monitoring are essential for the safety of the patient. Preoperative laboratory testing is advisable to learn the state of the whole body before anesthesia is administered. Intravenous fluids for circulatory support will speed the recovery of your patients, especially large dogs and older, possibly debilitated, pets. In addition to these precautions, it is a good idea to place an artificial tear ointment in the eyes to protect them and to cover both eyes to prevent foreign objects, such as calculus and bacteria, from lodging in the eyes. Steel treatment tables are cold and anesthesia lowers the body temperature as well. Support the core body temperature with insulated pads, blankets, or circulating water pads. Never use electrical heating pads because of the risk of burning the patient. To avoid the risk of calculus being aspirated, place gauze or paper towels at the back of the throat around the endotracheal tube. Do not forget to remove the packing at the end of the procedure.

Staff Safety

Precautions should be taken for the safety of the attending staff. These include anesthetic gas scavenging, safety glasses, a mask, and hair and hand protection. Dental X-rays should be held in place with film holders. The staff should stand a minimum of 6 feet away from the tube head of a dental X-ray machine to avoid exposure to scatter radiation. Use an X-ray monitoring service and badges to track staff exposure to radiation.

Patient Appearance

The animal should be as clean or cleaner when it is released than it was when it was admitted. Because dentistry can produce bleeding, the coat and mouth should be washed free of bloody discharge and the eyes should be wiped clean. Catheters should be removed and the haircoat cleaned and brushed. As a public relations touch, a little perfumed spray enhances the pet's appearance.

Home Care Instructions

Your veterinary technician can be an asset to your practice in the area of client education. Incorporating owner-delivered home teeth brushing is an important aspect of total dental care. A client who is willing to learn to brush the pet's teeth can maintain the pet's oral health and increase the interval between professional care visits. Your technician can demonstrate home care treatments and teeth brushing and explain the use of prescriptions and dental products. It is also a good idea to supply written instructions to reinforce those that are given orally. Clients may be feeling anxiety and stress about their pet's health and they may not comprehend or absorb all that is communicated to them. Written instructions allow your clients to review your instructions in a more relaxed environment. Some computer software systems allow home care instructions to be incorporated in the invoice. (See Chapter 7, Figures 7-1 and 7-2 (pp. 77, 78) for examples of home care instructions for dogs and cats.) A copy of your instructions should be stored in the patient folder as evidence of the communication.

Recall, Recheck, and Reminder

Again, these are the 3Rs of veterinary practice. A client should always leave the office with the next contact planned. A telephone callback should be scheduled for every patient that receives anesthesia. This shows your clients that you care about their pets. It also offers you or your staff the opportunity to answer questions and clarify treatment plans. Furthermore, it provides you with a chance to correct any problems that may arise. If the case is a major dental one, you will most likely want to schedule a recheck visit to monitor the healing process and success of home care efforts. Finally, the next dental examination should be scheduled and a reminder stored in your computer system or card file.

Referral Letters

If you begin accepting referrals for advanced level dental services, it is important to communicate with your referring colleague. Follow up your treatments with a phone call and letter describing the procedure and a note of thanks. Treat your referring veterinarian as you would wish to be treated. Avoid performing any extra services such as vaccinations, etc., that could easily be provided by the primary care veterinarian.

Feedback

Most of us would prefer to hear only positive feedback from our clients. We tend to become tense when a staff member communicates a problem about an upset client. However, always receiving positive feedback can give a false sense of security. Sometimes it takes negative feedback to keep us on our toes. Over time, I have come to understand that negative feedback is good, painful as it may have been at times. It is what allows a practice to learn about its problems and devise methods to correct

---

Golden Nugget

All feedback is beneficial and is important to seek.

---

them. Negative feedback can be a wonderful learning tool and can benefit your practice. I have the utmost respect for the client who will tell us when there is a problem, because it gives us the opportunity to turn a dissatisfied client into a satisfied client. This benefits the practice by stopping the spread of negative word-of-mouth and may even result in new referrals.

You can monitor the success of the dental health program by asking your clients for feedback. After the service has been performed, either the practitioner or a staff member should contact the client within the next one to three days to inquire about the pet's progress and the client's satisfaction with the service. Any doubts that you have about the importance of dental care will be dispelled once you begin to receive positive feedback from your clients. You will learn that providing dental care will improve the quality of life of the animals entrusted to your care. It won't take many cases for you to become a believer. As is often said in business management seminars, you must "walk the talk" to be successful in your efforts. Use the 3Rs to gather feedback.

Recalls

The best method for gathering feedback is your recall system. Use a computer callback feature to prompt phone calls to the client between 24 and 72 hours after the procedure. Most veterinary software packages have a program that will generate a telephone recall list. Depending on your own philosophy about the best timing for postoperative contact and the severity of the individual case, a telephone recall reminder should be generated between one and three days following the procedure. Index cards or phone lists on legal pads can be used in the absence of a computerized recall system. Staff members can perform this duty in routine cases. Let them be your ears and eyes and gather feedback for you. In more complex cases, a call from the veterinarian can make a tremendously positive impression on the client. Ask your client how the pet is doing following its dental procedure. And, please, *remember to listen* to the response!

▲   **Negative feedback:** If the patient is doing poorly or the client is dissatisfied, this gives the practice an opportunity to remedy the situation. If the pet is having difficulty with its postoperative recovery, you can schedule a recheck appointment and reevaluate its medical condition. Answer any questions or concerns that the client may have about the procedure or aftercare. It is important to be aware that the client is often feeling stress over the pet's procedure and may not remember all that is said when the animal is released. Often the client may misunderstand the instructions and administer the medication incorrectly. The sooner you are aware of a problem, the better your chance of changing a negative into a positive result.

▲   **Positive feedback:** When a client relates details of how well a pet is doing following a procedure, this information can serve to reinforce to the staff the value of the service. At our office, we hear stories nearly every day about old pets acting young again after major dental care. It is tremendously satisfying for the entire staff. It is easier to promote services when you believe that they are the right and best care you can give. Promote your success stories on your bulletin board and in your newsletters.

▲   **Assessment:** Evaluate the feedback and take action. Keep track of the results and monitor for patterns. Determine what your successful actions are and improve on them. You may find that you receive feedback about the pet's cleanliness or discomfort levels. Initiate corrective actions, if necessary. Learn from mistakes as well as from successes.

Recheck

For more invasive or complex cases, schedule recheck visits in one or two weeks. It is wise to monitor the healing process after oral surgery or extractions. The recheck visit will allow you to evaluate the progress of your patient and owner compliance and make adjustments in the treatment plan, if necessary. It is also another opportunity to ask for feedback.

Reminders

After receiving feedback, communicate with the client about scheduling the next visit. Let the client know when you think the pet will need to schedule its next periodic dental care and ask for verbal agreement. Each patient will have different dental needs. Annual dental cleanings will often be sufficient to maintain good dental health for most healthy companion animals.

Monitor Results

To gauge the success of your marketing program, it is important to measure your results and evaluate your successes and failures. The Marketing Program Result Sheet shown in Figure 8-1 leads us through the steps of accounting for the materials used and estimating profitability, using the Baseline Animal Hospital as an example. It is helpful to use a similar report sheet to determine a more accurate description of the costs of the individual marketing program and the production income earned. Figure 8-2 is a blank form for you to use with your own data.

Dr. Allright and his associate decided that their primary dental marketing program would take advantage of the National Pet Dental Health Month marketing program in February. They wrote a newsletter focusing on dental care and mailed it to

Date: February and March 1999

Problem: Only 200 (6%) of the patients received dental care in 1998. We would like to incorporate a dental program and increase the percentage of pets receiving dental care.

Goal: Increase the number of dental prophylaxes to 10% of the practice (300 cases) performed during 1999 for an average of 25 per month.

Project Design: Take advantage of the National Pet Dental Health Month and send newsletters focusing on dental care and send reminders to a selected group of owners and their pets.

Selection Criteria: We will send 300 dental reminder postcards in February and March to clients with pets over the age of 5 years that have never received dental care at this office. We will send additional cards on a monthly basis.

Income and Expenses of Project:	Amount
Clients/animals meeting criteria:	1,000 animals
Reminder cards mailed:	300 cards
Cost of reminder postcards: $.10 x 1,000	$100
Cost of mailing postcards: $.20 x 300	$60
Overhead cost of mailing reminders: 1 hr @ $1.50/minute	$90
Total costs of marketing program:	$250
Response: number of clients in February & March	60 prophylaxes 20% response rate
Average income: $150 per case	$9,000
Average variable expense: $18.82 per case	$1,129
Overhead expense: $767 per month x 2 months	$1,533
Veterinarian's salary: $30 per case	$1,800
Total cost of services:	$4,462
Plus the cost of the mailing:	$250
Total cost of marketing program & services:	$4,712
Contribution to return on investment:	$4,288

What Worked: We increased the number of dental prophylaxes beyond our stated goal of 25 per month. We performed 28 in February and 32 in March. The clients were very receptive and happy with the services. We were happy with the results and want to do more dentistry. The cost of the newsletter ($450 for printing and $400 bulk rate postage) was also offset by the increase in net income.

What Didn't Work: The staff wasn't used to performing so many dental cases and took longer than expected to complete the dental cleanings. The increased need for education and awareness helped us realize that we could expand but we lack the equipment and staff to handle a heavier caseload.

Suggestions for Next Time: Dr. Allright will attend the annual Veterinary Dental Forum in the fall and register for beginning dental seminars to increase his knowledge. He is interested in learning how to treat fractured teeth with root canal therapy. We will expand our equipment purchases and consider hiring another technician.

Figure 8-1   Baseline Animal Hospital Marketing Program Result Sheet.

Date:

Problem:

Goal:

Project Design:

Selection Criteria:

Income and Expenses of Project	Amount
Clients/animals meeting criteria:	
Reminder cards mailed:	
Cost of reminder postcards:	
Cost of mailing postcards:	
Overhead cost of mailing reminders:	
Total costs of marketing program:	
Response: number of clients	
Average income:	
Average variable expense:	
Overhead expense:	
Veterinarian's salary:	
Total cost of services:	
Plus the cost of the mailing:	
Total cost of marketing program & services:	
Contribution to return on investment:	

What Worked:

What Didn't Work:

Suggestions for Next Time:

Figure 8-2   Marketing Program Result Sheet.

Table 8-1   February–March Marketing Program Comparison of Results

	Before	**After**
Dental cases	32 animals	60 animals
Income	$3,200 ($100/case)	$9,000 ($150/case)
Total costs*	$2,774 ($86.70/case)	$4,460 ($74.34/case)
Net profit	$426	$4,540

*   This includes variable expenses ($18.82/case), overhead expense ($9,200/12 = $767/month), and veterinarian's 20-percent wage.

their entire clientele to increase awareness of the importance of dental care. They also selected a target group of pets over the age of five years that had never received dental care at their office. They assumed that most of these animals could benefit from dental care. Because they realized that they were not equipped to handle all of these cases, they decided to mail only a portion of the reminders each month.

The Marketing Program Result Sheet describes the results of the hospital's first dental program. This worksheet summarizes the results of the single marketing program that took place in February and March. The program performed very well. Compare the results of the marketing program in Table 8-1 to what the results might have been had Dr. Allright made no changes. Previously, each veterinarian performed an average of 8 dental cases a month. During the marketing program, they were able to increase this to an average of 15 per month. This number meets the lower end of the benchmark of 15–30 dental procedures per month suggested by Stephen Fischer, DVM.[2]

The Baseline Animal Hospital was contributing a small amount of profit on dental care prior to the implementation of the marketing program. By raising fees and nearly doubling the number of patients treated, the hospital was able to increase the contribution to profit more than tenfold. This was possible because overhead expense remained roughly the same ($9,200 per year or $767 per month) even though veterinarians' production income and expendables increased ($18.82 per case). The cost per case has decreased because the increased use of the dental department has spread the overhead expense over more cases, thus improving the productivity of the hospital.

The hypothetical results of dentistry and anesthesia combined are displayed in Table 8-3 (see page 92), showing an even more dramatic improvement in the bottom line. The numbers used for the Baseline Animal Hospital are shown to illustrate the impact that adding dental services can have on the bottom line of a practice. There will be a great variation between geographic areas and individual practices, but one fact will hold true: Dental services can be highly profitable for a practice to offer.

The Big Picture

At the end of each financial period, compare the most recent results with the previous or comparable period. You can measure results on a year-to-year comparison basis or by monthly or quarterly progression. By reviewing the statistics frequently, you can monitor the results of your efforts and make adjustments, as necessary, before small problems are compounded. If a program was successful, incorporate it into your regular service offering and marketing efforts. If your results were disappointing, analyze the feedback and implement corrections.

Collecting Data

Computerized veterinary software systems can provide a wealth of production statistics. Because veterinary medicine is cyclical in nature and there can be a wide variation in monthly production, quarterly data may give a truer picture of trends in the practice. It is helpful to maintain a spreadsheet of monthly data because it consolidates the key information into one worksheet that is easier to view. Compare data from one quarter to the performance of the previous quarter and compare your current data to the same period of last year. You will require three types of data to obtain a complete picture of your progress:

1. **Income data:** Collect financial data and total income figures from dental procedures. Compare this to previous periods. Analyze the changes and attempt to determine the reasons behind the differences.

2. **Expense data:** Determine the expenses related to the dental production from a profit and loss statement. Calculate the profitability of the dental department.

3. **Production data:** Compare the current production results with statistics from previous periods. Monitor the trends in your numbers, being aware of seasonal fluctuations due to such services as heartworm testing, flea programs, etc.

Golden Nugget

Increasing fees and volume while controlling expenses will result in greater net profit.

The Big Question

It is time to ask: "Is this profitable?" How is your progress toward the hospital's goals? Returning to the example of the Baseline Animal Hospital, we compare the results of the first full year of Dr. Allright's dental marketing program in Table 8-2. Overhead will change only slightly because it is constant and does not change appreciably with the volume of work performed. We assume that the hospital overhead per square foot increased by 2 percent, to $117.30, for cost-of-living inflation. Variable expenses increase with volume. When we consider the dental department by itself, the increase of 50 percent in the dental fees and the increase

Table 8-2   Baseline Animal Hospital Comparative Results

Statistic	Last Year	This Year	Percent Change
Number of dental cases	200	300	+50%
Average dental fee (excludes anesthesia, hospitalization, etc.)	$50	$75	+50%
Space for dental department	80 sq ft	80 sq ft	
Overhead/sq ft	$115.00	$117.30	
Income from dentistry	$10,000	$22,500	+125%
Direct dental expenses (estimate)	$500	$2,000	+300%
Overhead charged to dentistry	$9,200	$9,384	—
Total dental department expense	$9,700	$11,384	+5%
Net income from dentistry*	$300	$11,116	+3605%

* This excludes veterinarian's production income of 20 percent.

Table 8-3   Baseline Animal Hospital Combined Dental and Anesthesia Income

	Current Dentistry (in $)	Current Anesthesia (in $)	Current Combined (in $, at $150/case)	Previous Years Combined (in $, at $100/case)	$ Change (in $)
Income	22,500	22,500	45,000	20,000	25,000
Direct expenses	2,000 (estimated)	3,000 (300 cases @ $10)	5,000	2,500	1,500
Overhead	9,384	4,692	14,076	13,800	276
Total expenses	11,384	7,692	19,076	16,300	2,776
Net profit	11,116	14,808	25,924	3,400	22,524

in the number of cases increased the profitability of the hospital by approximately $11,000. In Table 8-3, anesthesia income is also added to the totals for a more comprehensive analysis.

The examples in Tables 8-2 and 8-3 show the potential profitability of high-quality dental care. By adding value to the services you offer your clients, you can justify charging a higher fee for your services. With the use of marketing tools, you can increase the volume of services performed. Developing a profitable dental department will allow you to elevate the quality and value of the hospital's services to a higher level and approach the goal of complete, quality health care for the whole pet.

The Final Step

It is time to fine tune your marketing plan and make adjustments. With the information you have gathered, review your marketing plan (see Chapter 3) and reassess each item. After analyzing the statistics and the feedback, determine what you might be able to do to improve. Ask questions of yourself, your staff, and your clientele. You can adjust your strategies as you go. If one of your strategies is having a negative impact, change or eliminate that strategy from your action plan. Do not allow the problem to compound itself. If a strategy is more successful than you anticipated, build on it and enhance the activity. Repeat the review process until you are satisfied with the results your practice has achieved. When you have accomplished the goals you established and are satisfied with the results, it is time to consider developing a new marketing plan that builds on your achievements.

Education

Do you wish to seek more education? Are you ready to learn more advanced dental techniques? Is there a need in your community for expanded services? Feedback from clients can be very helpful in determining needs in this area. If your clients are responding favorably to your dental program, consider expanding your services to include more advanced dental procedures.

Physical Plant

Is your dental operatory adequately designed and equipped to perform the level of service needed for increased volume? If there are problems with the layout, can the room be modified? If you have profits, consider purchasing additional equipment to expand your services.

Equipment and Supplies

Is your inventory adequate to perform your intended level of care? Establish order points and maintain adequate levels of supplies for increased production levels. Plan and budget for additional purchases and staffing when you expand your services.

Staff Training

Does your staff desire additional training? Can you or another clinician provide the training or do you need to seek outside training? Include the staff in your planning. It is important to involve them in the marketing program throughout the entire process. If they become an integral part of it, they will "sell" the value of dental care before you step into the exam room. When your staff believes in the services that your practice is offering and understands the fees, the promotion of dental services becomes easier. Once the dental department is well established, it will begin to build on its own merits. It is important to continue monitoring your performance, however, because lack of attention can lead to slippage and backsliding.

Fees and Marketing Strategies

Review each item in Chapter 7. Are your fees covering your expenses and contributing to your return on investment? Should you raise your fees? Are your clients complaining of "sticker shock"? If you are receiving negative feedback about your fees, the problem could be the method of presentation rather than the fees themselves. It may help to find a way to increase the "value" perceived by the client to make the fees more acceptable. Help your clients find a way to pay for your services by offering payment plans.

Implementation

Are you satisfied with the level of dental services that are being performed at your hospital? Can you and your staff do a better job? Do you have adequate staff to handle your increased workload? Consider adding a trained veterinary technician to your staff. Delegation is the key to an improved bottom line.[3]

Feedback

Always seek feedback. Keep asking questions. Listen and learn. Find out what is wrong and fix it. Learn what the practice is doing right and improve and expand upon it. Are your recall, recheck, and reminder systems in place and functioning well? Again, the 3Rs are your key source of feedback from your clients.

Fine Tune the Action Plan

Make the changes that are dictated by your analysis and repeat this process until you are satisfied with the results. It won't happen over night. Building a profitable dental department can be done successfully over a period of two to three years. Client acceptance takes time to evolve. As you improve your dental services, your clients will be learning the benefits of regular dental care for their pets. Success builds on itself. As you see the positive results of high-quality dental care, it will become easier for you to promote it to your clients. The rewards are healthy pets, satisfied pet owners, and a thriving practice.

Notes

1. E. R. Eisner, Personal conversations, December 1998.
2. S. C. Fisher, "Associates in Practice: Production Reports Provide Great Feedback," *DVM Newsmagazine* (December 1998): 46.
3. J. Rothstein, "Staff Leveraging Grows Talents, Profits," *Veterinary Product News* (April 1998): 26.

Sample Marketing Plan

Baseline Animal Hospital Dental Department Marketing Plan
January 1999

I. **Mission:** The mission of the Baseline Animal Hospital is to provide better dental services to the pets entrusted to our care so that they can continue to contribute to the lives of their owners by experiencing good health and long lives.

II. **Goals:** These are the goals of our hospital.

1. **Patient care:** We will impove the quality of the dental care delivered at our hospital.

2. **Finance:** We will increase the volume of dental care provided to improve our financial position.

3. **Facility and equipment:** We will expand the dental department of this hospital by purchasing the best equipment that we can afford to provide higher quality dental services.

4. **Education:** Our doctors and staff members will become more knowledgeable about dental health through continuing education courses and reading. We will encourage and support our staff to grow and develop to each individual's potential by financing continuing education courses.

5. **Marketing:** We will develop marketing tools to increase client awareness of dental health and promote dental services.

III. Market Analysis

Table A-1   Results of the SWOT Analysis for the Baseline Animal Hospital

Strengths	Weaknesses
▲ Good reputation in the community ▲ Strong interest in dentistry ▲ Well-trained, motivated staff ▲ Adequate facility, room to grow ▲ Newsletter in place ▲ Up-to-date computer system ▲ Some marketing experience ▲ Business has no outstanding loans	▲ Ultrasonic scaler broken ▲ Lack of dental expertise ▲ Lack of dental equipment ▲ Clientele uninformed about dental care ▲ Limited budget ▲ Profitability marginal: limited funds to develop dentistry
Opportunities	**Threats**
▲ Local economy strong ▲ Hospital is in a good location with good visibility ▲ Dental specialist in neighboring city ▲ Good standard of veterinary care in the community ▲ Clients are willing to pay above-average fees	▲ Local competition is strong ▲ Pet superstore within three miles, and it has a full-service hospital ▲ Local geographic area is stable, little opportunity for growth in client numbers

IV. **Objectives:** These are the objectives of the Baseline Animal Hospital.
  1. Educate the clientele about the importance of dental care.
  2. Provide above-average dental services beginning with dental prophylaxis.
  3. Perform a dental examination during every physical examination, whether the patient is well or ill.
  4. Schedule animals that have tartar buildup or inflamed gums for dental cleanings.
  5. Double the production volume for dental services in each of the next two years. This will increase dental income to 8 percent of total production income.
  6. Consider expanding dental services to endodontics and periodontics once basic services are well established.
  7. Budget $5,000 for continuing education, repairs, and purchases of dental equipment in each of the next two years. A dental X-ray machine (approximately $3,000) and a new moderately priced dental delivery system ($2,000–3,000) are at the top of the capital equipment wish list.

V. **Strategies:** These are the strategies that this hospital will pursue.
  1. Continuing education: Find basic level dental courses in the local area for veterinarians and technicians.
  2. Repair or replace existing dental equipment.
  3. Purchase new equipment for basic level dentistry.

4. Produce a newsletter focused on the importance of dental care.

5. Educate our clients about dental health during examination visits.

6. Add a dental reminder code to our reminder program.

7. Begin photographing dental cases for client education purposes.

8. Create a Smile Book of our success stories.

VI. **Action Plan**

1. **Continuing education:** Dr. Allright will attend the AAHA annual meeting this spring and attend the dental classes and a dental wet lab, if offered. He will also contact his personal dentist and investigate local continuing education opportunities. Finally, Dr. Allright will contact the board-certified veterinary dentist nearest to our practice and arrange to visit that practice to explore additional training. The associate veterinarian will also investigate local programs and attend meetings when possible. The deadline is January 30.

2. **Staff training:** The technicians will enroll at the AAHA annual meeting technician program in the spring and attend dental programs to improve their dental training. The deadline is January 30.

3. **Equipment:** To upgrade the hospital equipment, Dr. Allright and the technicians will tour the exhibit hall and investigate the purchase of dental equipment, specifically an ultrasonic scaler, polisher, and necessary supplies. They will also research the purchase of a dental X-ray machine at the AAHA annual meeting and through local X-ray equipment suppliers. The deadline is June 30 to purchase and install new equipment.

4. **Marketing efforts:** We will undertake the following marketing actions to improve client awareness of the importance of dental health and to increase the hospital income.

   a. The office manager will add a dental reminder to the computerized reminder system that will automatically send a reminder one year after dental care. This will be completed by January 15.

   b. The office manager will produce a newsletter highlighting the need for dental care. Our plan is to offer a dental health promotion for the slow month of September as a trial run and expand the program for National Pet Dental Health Month next February. The newsletter will be submitted to the printer by August l and mailed by August 25. The office manager will contact Hill's Pet Nutrition and their web site for promotional materials for National Pet Dental Health Month by October 30 for next February's newsletter.

   c. Dr. Allright will research the purchase of a camera or adapt his camera for close-up photography and begin taking photographs to use in a Smile Book. The deadline is April 30.

    d.   Beginning today, the entire staff will begin discussing the importance of dental care during each examination visit. We will schedule dental cleanings for all dogs and cats that have tartar build-up or inflamed gums.

VII. **Monitor results:** We will create a spreadsheet that will track the income from dental and anesthesia procedures and the numbers of various procedures. The spreadsheet will begin with last year's production reports to develop a basis for comparison. The deadline for the initial spreadsheet is February 28. The office manager will update the spreadsheet by the 10th of each month and present the summary to Dr. Allright. The results will be discussed at the next staff meeting after the 10th. We will evaluate the successes and failures and develop strategies to increase the probability of success of the dental marketing plan.

American Veterinary Dental College Suggested Reading Material

Although the following references are provided as suggested reading material for the AVDC examination, many of these sources are useful for additional information about the topics covered in this book. Much veterinary dental knowledge has been derived from human dentistry, and some of these sources are about the latter.

This reading list provided by the American Veterinary Dental College (October 1998).

Anusavice, K. J., *Phillips' Science of Dental Materials*, 10th ed. Philadelphia: W.B. Saunders, 1996.

Baum, L., R. W. Phillips, and M. R. Lind, *Textbook of Operative Dentistry*, 3d ed. Philadelphia: W.B. Saunders, 1995.

Carranza, F. A., and M. G. Newman, *Clinical Periodontology*, 8th ed. Philadelphia: W.B. Saunders, 1996.

Cohen, S., and R. C. Burns, *Pathways of the Pulp*, 7th ed. St. Louis: C. V. Mosby, 1998.

Crossley, D. A., and S. Penman, BSAVA, *Manual of Small Animal Dentistry*, 2d ed. Cheltenham, England: British Small Animal Veterinary Association, 1995.

Emily, P., and S. Penman, *Handbook of Small Animal Dentistry*, 2d ed. New York: Pergamon Press, 1994.

Evans, H. E., *Miller's Anatomy of the Dog*, 3d ed. Philadelphia: W.B. Saunders, 1993.

Frost, P., *Dentistry*. Veterinary Clinics of North America: Small Animal Practice, Philadelphia: W.B. Saunders, vol. 16(5). 1986.

Goaz, P. W., and S. C. White, *Oral Radiology—Principles and Interpretation*, 3rd ed. St. Louis: C. V. Mosby, 1994.

Gorrel, C., S. Penman, and P. Emily, *Handbook of Small Animal Oral Emergencies*. New York: Pergamon Press, 1993.

Harvey C. E., *Feline Dentistry.* Veterinary Clinics of North America: Small Animal Practice, vol. 22(6). Philadelphia: W.B. Saunders, 1992.

Harvey, C. E., *Veterinary Dentistry.* Philadelphia: W.B. Saunders, 1985.

Harvey, C. E., and P. Emily, *Small Animal Dentistry.* St. Louis: C. V. Mosby, 1993.

Holmstrom, S. E., *Canine Dentistry.* Veterinary Clinics of North America: Small Animal Practice, vol. 28(5). Philadelphia: W.B. Saunders, 1998.

Holmstrom, S. E., P. Frost, and E. R. Eisner, *Veterinary Dental Techniques,* 2d ed. Philadelphia: W.B. Saunders, 1998.

Journal of Veterinary Dentistry 7(1) (January1990) to present.

Kertesz, P. A., *A Colour Atlas of Veterinary Dentistry and Oral Surgery.* London: Wolfe, 1993.

Manfra-Marretta, S., *Dentistry: Problems in Veterinary Medicine.* Philadelphia: J. B. Lippincott, 1990.

Mulligan, T. W., M. S. Aller, and C. A. Williams, *Atlas of Canine and Feline Dental Radiography.* Trenton, N.J.: Veterinary Learning Systems, 1998.

Proffit, W.R., *Contemporary Orthodontics,* 2d ed. St. Louis: Mosby Year Book, 1993.

Rateitschak, K. H., et al., *Color Atlas of Dental Medicine—Periodontology,* 2d ed. New York: Thieme Medical Publishers, 1989.

Regezi, J. A., and J. Sciubba, *Oral Pathology—Clinical-Pathologic Correlations,* 2d ed. Philadelphia: W.B. Saunders, 1993.

Schroeder, H. E., *Oral Structural Biology.* New York: Thieme Medical Publishers, 1991.

Spodnick, G. J. (guest editor), "Veterinary Dentistry," *Seminars in Veterinary Medicine and Surgery (Small Animal)* 8(3). Philadelphia: W.B. Saunders, 1993.

Ten Cate, A. R., *Oral Histology: Development, Structure, and Function,* 4th ed. St. Louis: C. V. Mosby, 1994.

Thurmon, J. C., W. J. Tranquilli, and G. J. Benson, *Lumb & Jones' Veterinary Anesthesia,* 3d ed. Baltimore: Williams & Wilkins, 1996.

Wiggs, R. B., and H. B. Lobprise, *Veterinary Dentistry Principles and Practice.* Philadelphia: Lippincott-Raven, 1997.

Year Book of Dentistry®. St. Louis: Mosby Year Book: last five issues.

Other journals with valuable dental articles include the following:

▲   *Compendium on Continuing Education for the Practicing Veterinarian*

▲   *Compendium of Continuing Education in Dentistry*

▲   *Journal of the American Animal Hospital Association*

▲   *Journal of the American Veterinary Medical Association*

▲   *Veterinary Surgery*

Dental Manufacturers and Distributors List

3 M Dental Products Division
Bldg. 260-28-09
3M Center
St. Paul, MN 55144
(800) 634-2249
(612) 733-1110
FAX: (612) 733-9973
Products: Many dental products

Addison Biological Laboratory, Inc.
507 N. Cleveland Ave.
Fayette, MO 65248
(800) 331-2530
(660) 248-2215
FAX: (660) 248-2554
E-mail: alaborat@mail.coin.missouri.edu
Products: Home dental care products—
Maxi/Guard Gel

AFP Imaging Corporation
250 Clearbrook Rd.
Elmsford, NY 10523
(914) 592-6100
FAX (914) 592-6148
Web site: www.afpimaging.com
E-mail: ghelf@afpimaging.com
Products: Intraoral X-ray system

Aldrich/Girard Company
3625 N. Andrews Ave.
Oakland Park, FL 33309
(800) 654-5705
(954) 561-8597
FAX: (954) 563-1124
Products: Electric motor-driven
handpieces, nitrogen air-driven dental
equipment, air scalers, ultrasonic scalers

Allerderm, Inc.
P.O. Box 162059
Ft. Worth, TX 76161
(800) 338-3659
FAX: (817) 831-8327
Products: Professional prophylactic and
home care dental products

Analytic Technology Corp.
15233 Northeast 90th St.
Redmond, WA 98052
(800) 428-2808
(206) 883-2445
FAX: (206) 882-3128
Products: Touch 'n heat, apex locator,
other dental products

This listing is not all-inclusive. The author has made every attempt to include all manufacturers and distributors of veterinary dental equipment. This listing is current as of August 1999.

Arista Surgical Supply, Inc.
67 Lexington Ave.
New York, NY 10010
(800) 223-1984
(212) 679-3694
FAX: (212) 696-9046
Products: Dental and surgical instruments

Aseptico, Inc.
19501-144th Ave. Northeast
Suite B-400
Woodinville, WA 98072
(800) 425-5913
(206) 487-2808
FAX: (206) 487-2808
Products: Dental supplies and equipment

ASVDT (American Society of Veterinary Dental Technicians)
316 Shore Rd.
Venice, FL 34285
(941) 488-7802
FAX: (941) 484-1439
Product: Society membership

AVLS
P.O. Box 67127
Lincoln, NE 68506
(800) 444-3634
FAX: (402) 466-3501
Products: Client education aids

Brasseler USA, Inc.
800 King George Blvd.
Savannah, GA 31419
(800) 841-4222
(912) 925-8525
FAX: (912) 927-8671
Products: Burs, files, diamonds,
instruments

Burns Veterinary Supply
Nationwide Office
1900 Diplomat Dr.
Farmers Branch, TX 75234
(800) 922-8767
(972) 620-9941
FAX: (972) 620-1071
Products: Veterinary distributor of dental
products and equipment

Butler Company
5000 Bradeton Ave.
Dublin, OH 43017
(800) 848-5983
(614) 761-9095
FAX: (614) 761-9096
Products: Complete veterinary supply
distributor of dental products and
equipment

Cameron-Miller, Inc.
3949 South Racine Ave.
Chicago, IL 60609
(800) 621-0142
(312) 523-6360
FAX: (312) 523-9495
Products: Electrosurgery equipment

C.D.M.V. Inc.
C.P. 608.2999 Choquette
St. Hyancinthe
Quebec, Canada J25 7C2
(514) 773-6073
FAX: (514) 773-4370
Products: Complete veterinary supply
distributor of dental products and
equipment

Centrix, Inc.
770 River Rd.
Shelton, CT 06484
(800) 235-5862
(203) 929-5582
FAX: (203) 929-6804
Products: Centrix syringe, bonding agents

Cislak Manufacturing, Inc.
1866 Johns Dr.
Glenview, IL 60025
(800) 239-2904
(847) 239-2904
FAX: (847) 729-2994
Products: Hand instruments, feline elevator kit, sharpening aids, full-service dental supplier

Colgate Oral Pharmaceuticals
One Colgate Way
Canton, MA 02021
(800) 225-3756
(617) 821-2880
FAX: (617) 828-7330
Products: Viadent mouthwash and gingival flush

Coltene/Whaledent
750 Corporate Dr.
Mahwah, NJ 07430
(800) 221-3046
(201) 512-8000
FAX: (201) 529-2103
Products: Parapulpar pins and endodontic posts, hand instruments

Confi-Dental Products Company
416 South Taylor Ave.
Louisville, CO 80027
(800) 383-5158
(303) 665-7535
FAX: (303) 666-4320
Products: Glass ionomer and composite restorative materials

Cosmedent, Inc.
5419 North Sheridan Rd.
Chicago, IL 60640
(800) 621-6729
(312) 989-6844
FAX: (312) 989-1826
Products: Cements, composites, hybrids, instruments, polishing discs, polishing strips, cups, points, polishing pastes

Den Mat Corporation
2727 Skyway Dr.
Santa Maria, CA 93456
(800) 433-6628
(805) 922-8491
FAX: (805) 922-6933
Products: Restorative products, bonding agents, composites, glass ionomers

Dentalaire
17165 Newhope St., Ste J
Fountain Valley, CA 92708
(800) 866-6881
(714) 540-9969
FAX: (714) 540-9947
Products: Air compressors, complete line of dental supplies, handpiece repair

Dental Enterprises
1976 South Bannock St.
Denver, CO 80223
(800) 466-1466
(303) 777-6717
FAX: (303) 777-6726
Products: Complete line of new and used dental equipment. Service of equipment and handpieces.

Dentsply International
570 West College Ave.
P.O. Box 872
York, PA 17405
(800) 877-0020
(717) 845-7511
FAX: (717) 849-4376
Products: Scalers, infection control paste

Dentsply/Gendex Division
4379 S. Howell Ave., Ste #2
Milwaukee, WI 53207
(800) 769-2909
(414) 769-2888
FAX: (414) 769-2868
Products: Dental radiograph machines and processors

Dentsply/Rinn Division
1212 Abbott Dr.
Elgin, IL 60123
FAX: (800) 544-0787
Products: Radiographic supplies

Dr. Shipp's Dental Laboratory
351 North Foothill Rd.
Beverly Hills, CA 90210
(310) 550-0107
FAX: (310) 550-1664
Products: Dental models and full-service dental supplies

Eastman Kodak Company
HSD/Dental Products
343 State St.
Rochester, NY 14650
(800) 933-8031
(716) 724- 5631
FAX: (716) 724-5797
Products: Intraoral and panoramic radiographic film and supplies

Easy Tray, Inc.
2209 North 56th
Seattle, WA 98103
(800) 726-1628
(206) 545-7971
FAX: (206) 545-8011
Products: Custom trays

Ellman International, Inc.
1135 Railroad Ave.
Hewlett, NY 11557
(516) 569-1482
FAX: (516) 569-0054
Products: Radiosurgical instruments, nylon and metal splint material

Engler Engineering Corp.
1099 E. 47th St.
Hialeah, FL 33013-2194
(800) 445-8581
FAX: (305) 685-7671
E-mail: infor@engler-engineering.com
Web site: www.engler-engineering.com
Products: Ultrasonic scaler/polishers

Espe America
1710 Romano Dr.
P.O. Box 111
Norristown, PA 19404
(800) 344-8235
(800) 548-3987
(610) 277-3800
FAX: (610) 239-2301
Products: Restorative material

Fort Dodge Laboratories
800 Fifth St. N.W.
Fort Dodge, IA 50501
(800) 383-6343
(515) 955-4600
FAX: (800) 846-8626
Products: Nolvadent antimicrobial dentifrice, Torbugesic SA, Torbutrol

Friskies Petcare Co.
800 N. Brand Blvd.
Glendale, CA 91203
(818) 543-7749
FAX: (818) 549-6509
Products: Chew-eez

GC America, Inc.
3737 West 127th St.
Alsip, IL 60803
(800) 323-7063
(708) 597-0900
FAX: (708) 371-5103
Products: Dental cements, restorative materials (Fuji)

George Taub-Products
277 New York Ave.
Jersey City, NJ 07307
(800) 828-2634
(201) 798-5353
FAX: (201) 659-7186
Products: Dental products

Heinz Pet Products
One Riverfront Place
Newport, KY 41071
(606) 655-5042
Products: Educational dental booklet, dental home care products

Henry Schein Inc.
135 Duryea Rd.
Melville, NY 11747
(800) 872-4346
(516) 843-5500
FAX: (516) 843-5696
Products: Complete supply of veterinary and dental products

Heska Corporation
1825 Sharp Point Dr.
Ft. Collins, CO 80525
(970) 493-7272
FAX: (970) 221-2392
Web site: www.heska.com
Products: Perioceutics, sensor devices, pulse oximeters, clinical pathology

Hill's Pet Nutrition, Inc.
P.O. Box 148
Topeka, KS 66601
(800) 354-4557
(913) 354-8523
FAX: (800) 442-9910
Web site: www.hillspet.com
Products: Dog and cat food beneficial to dental hygiene

Hu-Friedy Mfg. Co., Inc.
3232 N. Rockwell St.
Chicago, IL 60618
(800) 483-7433
(312) 975-6100
FAX: (312) 975-1683
Products: Scalers, probes, dental instruments

I DE-Interstate Dental, Inc.
1500 New Horizons Blvd.
Amityville, NY 11701
(800) 666-8100
(516) 957-8300
FAX: (516) 957-5781
Products: Dental materials, pharmaceuticals

IDEXX Laboratories
One IDEXX Dr.
Westbrook, ME 04092
(800) 551-0998
FAX: (207) 856-0625
Products: Laboratory equipment

iM3, Inc.
12013 NE 99th St., Suite 1670
Vancouver, WA 98683
(360) 254-2981
FAX: (360) 254-2940
E-mail: imthree@pacifier.com
Web site: www.im3vet.com
Products: Air driven dental system

Image Imprints
P.O. Box 1029
North Hampton, MA 01061
(413) 586-4439
FAX: (413) 586-4439
Products: Imprinted toothbrushes

Innovative Technology Sales
149 John Deese Dr.
Ft. Collins, CO 80524
(970) 482-9077
FAX: (970) 484-1618
Products: Portident Tabletop Dental System

Jansen Pharmaceuticals
1125 Trenton-Harbourtin Rd.
P.O. Box 200
Titusville, NJ 08560
(800) 526-7763
(609) 730-2000
FAX: (609) 730-2461
Products: Fentanyl patch (Duragesic)

JB Lippincott Publishing
2227 East Washington Sq.
Philadelphia, PA 19106
(215) 238-4200
FAX: (215) 238-4227
Products: Dental texts

JEM Systems
14550 E. Easter Ave., Ste. 1000
Englewood, CO 80112
(800) 203-5406
(303) 766-0376
FAX: (303) 766-8584
Products: Delivery systems, compressors, radiograph units, burs, handpieces, hand instruments

J. Morita USA, Inc.
14712 Bentley Cir.
Tustin, CA 92780
(800) 752-9729
(714) 544-2854
FAX: (714) 730-1048
Products: Composite resins, dental adhesives, restorative materials, X-ray machines, video imaging system

Johnson & Johnson Dental Products Division
1 Johnson and Johnson Place
New Brunswick, NJ 08933
(800) 526-3967
(908) 524-0400
FAX: (908) 874-2545
Products: Surgicel

Jorgensen Laboratories, Inc.
1450 N. VanBuren Ave.
Loveland, CO 80538
(970) 669-2500
FAX: (970) 663-5042
Products: Dental instruments

Kerr Corporation
28200 Wick Rd.
Romulus, MI 48174
(800) 537-7123
(714) 516-7633
Products: Composites, impression material, amalgam, laboratory products, endodontic instruments

Lares Research, Inc.
295 Lockhead Ave.
Chico, CA 96973
(800) 347-3289
FAX: (916) 345-1870
Products: Handpieces

L.D. Caulk/Dentsply
Lakeview and Clark Aves.
Milford, DE 19963
(800) 532-2855
(302) 422-4511
Products: Composite restoratives, bases, liners, cements, amalgam restoratives, impression materials

Lifelearn
MacNabb House
University of Guelph
Ontario, Canada NIG 2W1
(800) 375-7994
FAX: (519) 767-1101
Products: Audiovisual dental educational materials

Macan Engineering & Mfg. Co.
1564 North Damen Ave.
Chicago, IL 60622
(773) 772-2000
FAX: (773) 772-2003
Products: Electrosurgery equipment

Masel Inc.
2701 Partram Rd.
Bristol, PA 19007
(800) 423-8227
(215) 785-1600
FAX: (215) 785-1680
Products: Orthodontic instruments, materials, wire splinting products

Matrix Medical, Inc.
145 Mid County Dr.
Orchard Park, NY 14127
(800) 847-1000
(716) 662-6550
FAX: (716) 662-7130
Products: Dental compressors, anesthesia, emergency care products

Medidentia
39-23 62nd St.
P.O. Box 409
Woodside, NY 11377
(800) 221-0750
(718) 672-4670
FAX: (718) 672-4670
Products: Endodontic instruments, handpieces

MedRx Inc™
13800 Park Blvd.
Seminole, FL 33776
(888) 392-1234
FAX: (813) 392-9256
Web site: www.medrx-use.com
Products: Endoscopic instruments, intraoral camera

Midwest Dental Products Corp.
901 West Oakton St.
Des Plaines, IL 60018
(800) 800-7202
(847) 640-4800
FAX: (847) 640-6165
Products: Electric delivery systems, handpieces, and burs

Miltex Instrument Co., Inc.
6 Ohio Dr.-CB 5006
Lake Success, NY 11042
(800) 645-8000
(516) 775-7100
FAX: (516) 775-7185
Products: Hand instruments, burs, extraction forceps

Minxray
3611 Commercial Ave.
Northbrook, IL 60062
(800) 221-2245
(847) 564-0323
FAX: (847) 564-9040
Products: Portable radiographic equipment

Nephron Corporation
P.O. Box 1974
321 East 25th St.
Tacoma, WA 98401
(800) 426-3603
(206) 383-1002
FAX: (206) 383-2751
Products: Hand instruments and dental products

Nutramax Laboratories, Inc.
5024 Campbell Blvd., Ste B
Baltimore, MD 21236
(800) 925-5187
FAX: (800) 925-0361 or (410) 931-4009
Web site: www.nutramaxlabs.com
Products: Consil™, a synthetic bone graft material; Cosequin®

Nylabone Products
P.O. Box 427
Neptune, NJ 07753
(800) 631-2188
(201) 988-8400
FAX: (908) 988-5466
Products: Home care chewing aids

Omni Products
P.O. Box 762
Bountiful, UT 84011
(800) 777-2972
(801) 298-7663
FAX: (801) 298-2984
Products: Diamond burs

Omni Products International
P.O. Box 100
Gravette, AR 72736
(800) 284-4123
(501) 787-5232
FAX: (501) 787-5516
Products: Fluoride gels, rinses, toothbrushes, implants

Orascoptic Research, Inc.
5225-3 Verona Rd., Bldg. 3
P.O. Box 44451
Madison, WI 53744-4451
(608) 278-0111
FAX: (608) 278-0101
Products: BodyGuard Seating System
(loupes, lights, stools), zeon illuminator

Oxyfresh USA, Inc.
East 12928 Indiana Ave.
Spokane, WA 99220
(800) 333-7374
(509) 924-4999
FAX: (509) 924-5285
Products: Home care products

Pascal Company, Inc.
2929 Northeast Northrup Way
Bellevue, WA 98004
(800) 426-8051
(206) 827-4694
FAX: (206) 827-6893
Products: Dental products

Patterson Dental Company
1031 Mendota Heights Rd.
St. Paul, MN 55120
(800) 328-5536
(612) 686-1600
FAX: (612) 686-9331
Products: Dental supplies

Pearson Dental
13847 Delsur St.
San Fernando, CA 91340
(800) 535-4535
(818) 362-2600
Products: Vibrators, amalgamators, dental
materials, equipment, supplies

Periogiene Woodall and Associates
3188 Airway Ave.
Costa Mesa, CA 92626
(800) 368-5776; (714) 662-3300
FAX: (888) 368-4787
Products: Odontoson scaler

Pets Veterinary Dental Laboratory
803 W. College Ave.
P.O. Box 867
Waukesha, WI 53187
(800) 558-7734
(414) 542-5100
FAX: (414) 542-1717
Products: Full-service dental laboratory

Pfizer
812 Springdale Dr.
Exton, PA 19341
(800) 733-5500
(610) 363-3100
FAX: (800) 228-5176
Web site: www.pfizer.com/ah
Products: Clavamox (antibiotic)

Pharmacia & Upjohn
7000 Portage Rd.
Kalamazoo, MI 49001
(800) 253-8600 x32404 [tech. services]
(616) 833-2404
FAX: (616) 833-3305
Products: Antirobe (antibiotic), client
home care education and office visual
aids

Precision Ceramics Dental Laboratory
9591 Central Ave.
Montclair, CA 91763
(800) 223-6322
Products: Full-service dental laboratory

Pro-Dentec
633 Lawrence St.
Batesville, AR 72503
(800) 228-5595
(501) 698-2300
FAX: (501) 793-5554
Products: WHO (World Health
Organization) sensor probe

Ribbond Inc.
1326 5th Ave., Ste 640
Seattle, WA 98101
(800) 624-4554
(206) 340-8870
FAX: (206) 382-9354
Product: Splinting material

Richmond Dental Company
P.O. Box 34276
Charlotte, NC 28234
(800) 277-0377
(704) 376-0380
FAX: (704) 342-1892
Products: Cotton pellets and products

Roth International Ltd.
669 West Ohio St.
Chicago, IL 60610
(800) 445-0572
(312) 733-1478
FAX: (312) 733-7398
Products: Endodontic sealers

Rx Honing Machine Corp.
1301 East Fifth St.
Mishawaka, IN 46544
(800) 346-6464
(219) 259-1606
FAX: (219) 259-9163
Products: Sharpening equipment

Shofu Dental Corporation
4025 Bohanon Dr.
Menlo Park, CA 94025
(800) 827-4638
(415) 324-0085
FAX: (415) 323-3180
Products: Glass ionomers

SS White/Burs, Inc.
1145 Towbin Ave.
Lakewood, NJ 08701
(800) 535-2877
(732) 905-1100
FAX: (732) 905-0987
Products: Burs

Shor-Line/Schoer Manufacturing Co.
2221 Campbell St.
Kansas City, MO 64108
(800) 444-1579
(816) 471-0488
FAX: (816) 471-5339
Products: Scalers, compressors, treatment tables

Siemens/Pelton & Crane
11727 Fruehauf Dr.
Charlotte, NC 28273
(800) 659-6560
(704) 523-3212
FAX: (704) 588-5770
Products: Sterilizers

Silverman's Dental
22 Industrial Park Dr.
Port Washington, NY 11050
(800) 448-3384
(516) 484-7660
FAX: (516) 484-7645
Products: Distributes general dental supplies and equipment through Henry Schein, Inc.

Sontec Instruments
7248 S. Tucson Way
Englewood, CO 80112
(800) 821-7496
(303) 790-9411
FAX: (303) 792-2606
Products: Surgical instruments

Spartan USA, Inc.
1727 Larkin Williams Rd.
Fenton, MO 63026
(800) 325-9027
(314) 343-8300
FAX: (314) 343-5794
Products: Piezo scalers

St. Jon Laboratories
1656 West 240th St.
Harbor City, CA 90710
(800) 969-7387
(310) 326-2720
FAX: (310) 326-8026
Products: VRx toothpastes and home care products, fluoride foam, toothbrushes

Star Dental Products
1816 Colonial Village Lane
Lancaster, PA 17601
(800) 422-7827
(717) 291-1161
FAX: (717) 291-3249
Products: Titan-S scaler, handpieces, ultrasonic equipment

Suburban Surgical Co., Inc.
275 Twelfth St.
Wheeling, IL 60090
(800) 323-7366
(708) 537-9320
Products: Compressors, handpieces, treatment tables

Sullivan Dental Products, Inc.
10920 W. Lincoln Ave.
West Allis, WI 53227
(800) 558-5200
(414) 321-8881
FAX: (414) 321-8865
Products: Scalers, anesthetic infection control

Summit Hill Laboratories
P.O. Box 535
Navesink, NJ 07752
(800) 922-0722
(201) 291-3600
Products: Scalers, electrosurgery units, anesthetic machines

SurgiTel/General Scientific Corp.
77 Enterprise Dr.
Ann Arbor, MI 48103
(313) 996-9200
FAX: (313) 662-0520
Products: Magnification loupes and light systems

Teledyne-Getz
1550 Greenleaf Ave.
Elk Grove Village, IL 60007
(800) 323-6650
(312) 593-3334
Products: Alginate, cements, trays, light cure materials, surgical dressing, prophy cups

Temerex
112 Albany Ave.
P.O. Box 182
Freeport, NY 11520
(800) 645-1226
(516) 868-6221
FAX: (516) 868-5700
Products: Cements, bleaching etchants

Thermafil
5001 East 68th St.
Tulsa, OK 74136
(800) 662-1202
(918) 493- 6598
FAX: (800) 597-2779
Products: Warm gutta percha products

THM Biomedical, Inc.
325 South Lake Ave.
Duluth, MN 55804
(800) 327-6895
(218) 720-3628
FAX: (218) 720-3715
Product: Polylactic acid granules®

Tulsa Dental Products
5001 East 68th St., Ste 500
Tulsa, OK 74136
(800) 662-1202
(918) 493-6598
FAX: (918) 493-6599
Products: Endodontic materials and
supplies: Thermafil, Profile 29 files

**Veterinary Dental Laboratory of
America**
7733 Main St.
Fairview, PA 16415
(814) 474-5806
Products: Fabricated orthodontic
appliances and restoratives

Veterinary Medicine Publishing Co.
9073 Lenexa Dr.
Lenexa, KS 66215
(800) 255-6864
(913) 492-4300
FAX: (913) 492-4157
Web site: www.vetmedpub.com
Products: Veterinary dental books and
journals

Vetoquinol U.S.A., Inc., ImmunoVet
5910-G Breckenridge Pkwy.
Tampa, FL 33610
(813) 621-9447
FAX: (813) 621-0751
Products: Stomadhex™, bioadhesive patch

Vetko
4931 North Park Dr.
Colorado Springs, CO
(719) 598-8782
Products: Ultrasonic scaler, circulating hot
water pad

Vident
3150 East Birch St.
Brea, CA 92621
(800) 828-3839
(714) 961-6200
FAX: (714) 961-6299
Products: Inceram indirect restoratives

VRx® Pharmaceuticals
See St. Jon Laboratories

X-Ray Innovations
6325 Eaton St.
Hollywood, FL 33024
(954) 986-2334
FAX: (954) 986-2334
Products: Portable prophy table

W.B. Saunders Co.
Independence Square West
Philadelphia, PA 19106
(215) 238-7832
FAX: (215) 238-8483
Products: Medical publications

Welch Allyn Dental Systems
4619 Jordan Rd.
P.O. Box 187
Skaneateles Falls, NY 13153
(800) 867-3832
(315) 685-9514
FAX: (315) 685-7905
Products: Cameras, lights

Whaledent International
236 5th Ave.
New York, NY 10001
(800) 221-3046
(212) 696-8000
FAX: (212) 532-1644
Products: Dental supplies, endodontic
instruments, electrosurgical equipment

Young Dental
13705 Shoreline Court East
Earth City, MO 63045
(800) 325-1881
(314) 344-0010
FAX: (314) 344-0021
Products: Prophy paste, fluoride,
instruments

Index

Note: *f.* after a page number indicates a figure; *t.* indicates a table.

About the Author

Coralee Eisner, CVT, MBA, is the practice manager at the Campus Veterinary Clinic, PC, in Denver, Colorado, an AAHA-accredited hospital since 1973. She has been involved in veterinary medicine as a technician and practice manager for more than 20 years, applying her business background to veterinary practice management. As a lifelong resident of Colorado, she attended Colorado State University, earning a bachelor's degree in economics. After college, Ms. Eisner worked as a statistician and computer programmer for Standard and Poor's, a subsidiary of McGraw-Hill 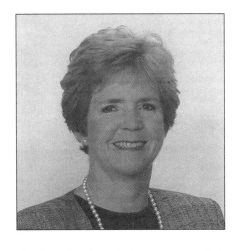 Publishing Company. After meeting her future husband, Edward Eisner, DVM, Dipl. AVDC, she became interested in veterinary medicine. She earned an associate's degree from Bel-Rea Institute of Animal Technology, followed by a master's degree in business administration from the University of Colorado.

Ms. Eisner lives in Littleton, Colorado, with her husband and daughter. The family includes a Labrador Retriever and two cats.